HEALTHCARE EXECUTIVES

The Essentials for Excellence in Leadership and Management

Professor Dirk Pickuth
MD, PhD, MDs (honoris causa)

COPYRIGHT

Matador
9 Priory Business Park, Wistow Road,
Kibworth Beauchamp, Leicestershire. LE8 0RX
Tel: 0116 279 2299
Email: books@troubador.co.uk
Web: www.troubador.co.uk/matador
Twitter: @matadorbooks

ISBN 978 1789017 069

British Library Cataloguing in Publication Data.
A catalogue record for this book is available from the British Library.

Printed and bound in the UK by TJ International, Padstow, Cornwall

Matador is an imprint of Troubador Publishing Ltd

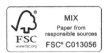

To Britain — my wellspring of happiness.

In aid of

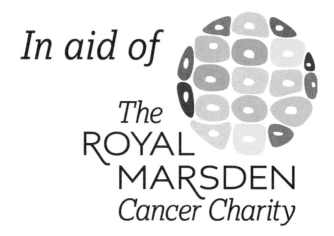

The
ROYAL
MARSDEN
Cancer Charity

Registered Charity Number: 1095197

I will be donating all royalties of the book to The Royal Marsden Cancer Charity.

The Royal Marsden Cancer Charity raises money solely to support The Royal Marsden, a world-leading cancer centre.

The donations will help The Royal Marsden ensure their nurses, doctors and research teams can provide the very best care and develop life-saving treatments, which are used across the UK and around the world.

Thank you for your support of 'Healthcare Executives – The Essentials for Excellence in Leadership and Management' and The Royal Marsden Cancer Charity.

Professor Dirk Pickuth MD, PhD, MDs (honoris causa)

The Royal Marsden Cancer Charity is very grateful for Professor Pickuth's support as we continue to look for ways to improve the lives of people affected by cancer.

Edwin Drummond
Head of Individual and Corporate Philanthropy
The Royal Marsden Cancer Charity
London, United Kingdom

CONTENTS

ABOUT THE CONCEPT

Short synopsis: The book is a powerful guide for healthcare professionals from all backgrounds and at every level. Featuring a high degree of conciseness, practicality and comprehensiveness, the book is a capability framework that aims to encourage, inspire and enlighten future and current healthcare leaders and managers.

Key words: Healthcare | leadership | management | excellence | career | essentials

Key features: Succinct text | fact boxes | bullet format | quick reference | expert insights | practical tips

Target audience: Future and current healthcare leaders and managers

Typical readership: Medical Directors | Clinical Directors | Consultants | Doctors | Chief Executives | Board Chairs | Nurses | Policymakers | Plus other healthcare professionals and experts at various levels

ABOUT THE BOOK

Effective and sustainable leadership and management are vitally important to care quality and health outcomes.

This handy, authoritative and inspiring book provides a highly systematic and practical overview of the knowledge, skills and behaviours required for effective healthcare leadership and management. It covers all key topics and recent developments, with a focus on high quality care and best practice.

The author presents the material concisely and precisely, walking the reader through all important aspects of leadership and management within today's complex healthcare environment, with special attention to situations and examples in the United Kingdom.

Keeping busy executives in mind, the text is streamlined with fact boxes, bullet point summaries and smart graphics to allow rapid and easy reading, while providing quick reference through chapter overviews and descriptive headlines. There are hundreds of useful and actionable tips and hints for aspiring and current healthcare leaders and managers.

Value and outcomes for patients are the main goals of a healthcare organisation. The book advocates an adaptive, forward-focused, value-based, outcome-oriented, collective leadership and management style. It aims to increase reader knowledge, raise effectiveness, improve performance and advance healthcare careers. As such, it is an indispensable guide to mastering the key elements of leadership and management for all those who wish to improve their productivity and maximise their impact.

Typical challenges faced in healthcare do not have national boundaries, nor do they have national solutions. As an eminent Medical Director at a large healthcare trust for more than a decade, author Professor Dirk Pickuth is a senior healthcare leader with extensive experience in healthcare leadership and management. He is an advocate of the British National Health Service (NHS) which has been judged by many sources as the best, most affordable and safest healthcare system in the world. Grounded in the author's international expertise, the book takes a universal perspective and is a valuable resource for anyone involved in the healthcare sector around the world.

Professor Pickuth has enjoyed a long and successful career as an international healthcare leader. He is a trust executive with an outstanding and unblemished track record of delivering change. Sharing his expertise, insights and wisdom, Professor Pickuth reveals the methods and techniques he applies in providing a comprehensive framework of leadership excellence and management efficiency.

The reader will learn how to apply in practice the principles of outstanding performance on both a personal and a professional level. This is the definitive guide for those wishing to move to game changing action in healthcare leadership and management.

ABOUT THE AUTHOR

Professor Dirk Pickuth MD, PhD, MDs (honoris causa)

- Medical Director of the Caritas Hospital Foundation Trust, Saarbrücken, Germany
- Head of the Department of Radiology at the Caritas Academic Teaching Hospital, Saarbrücken, Germany
- Medical studies in Kiel, London and Edinburgh | Clinical Research Fellow at the Royal Marsden Hospital | Radiology training at Heidelberg University | Professor of Radiology | Honorary Professor of Imaging Techniques and Medical Physics | Visiting Professor at the University of East Anglia in Norwich
- Member of the Royal College of Radiologists | Member of the British Institute of Radiology | Member of the Faculty of Medical Leadership and Management

For over two decades, Professor Dirk Pickuth has been a visionary in the leadership development field, serving as a trust leader and change manager. He advocates a high performance culture and practises evidence based leadership, holding a respected role in engaging staff, empowering people and building trust. With a reputation for excellence in areas such as interpersonal skills, communication style and team working, Professor Pickuth sets the tone for an environment that encourages highly motivated staff to more readily act in the best interests of their patients and consistently observe the highest professional standards in clinical care.

As Medical Director of the Caritas Hospital Foundation Trust in Saarbrücken, Germany, since 2006, Executive Director and a full voting member of the Trust's Executive Board, Professor Pickuth holds a flagship role in contributing to the development of the trust's strategy from both an expert medical and a broader business perspective. Since 2001 he has also served as the Head of the Department of Diagnostic and Interventional Radiology at the Caritas Academic Teaching Hospital. The Caritas Hospital Foundation Trust is recognised as one of the best performing healthcare trusts in Germany.

From 1991 to 1992, Professor Pickuth studied medicine in London and Edinburgh and was a Clinical Research Fellow at the Royal Marsden Hospital and the Institute of Cancer Research in London. His professional affiliations include membership of the Royal College of Radiologists and the British Institute of Radiology since 1996. Since then he has shared in many successful cooperative activities with British colleagues in clinical, scientific and management areas. His times in the United Kingdom have included intensive travel throughout the whole country, while cultivating a rich network of great friends and acquaintances, both personal and professional.

Professor Pickuth's experiences of living and working in the United Kingdom alongside people from a wide variety of backgrounds and cultures impressed and influenced him deeply. His affinity for Britain and the National Health Service (NHS) stems from a passionate appreciation of the great traditions of healthcare excellence, academic research and clinical teaching in British medicine.

As a way to express his gratitude for the cumulative influence of the United Kingdom on his life, he dedicated his bestselling radiology textbook *Klinische Radiologie Fakten [Clinical Radiology Facts]* to the British people.

Currently at the Caritas Hospital Foundation Trust in Saarbrücken, Professor Pickuth works in close collaboration with the Chief Executive Officer, Chief Operating Officer and Chief Nursing Officer to ensure that a clear and coherent medical strategy is developed and translated into service improvements. He is an eminent adviser on medical issues, clinical governance matters and care quality. As the responsible medical expert, he leads daily operations in providing excellence in patient safety, clinical effectiveness and patient experience in an environment where the best care is offered in a timely, consistent and reliable manner.

In his activities in leading patient centred care through effective role modelling and continuous professional development of all medical staff, Professor Pickuth fosters and nurtures constructive working relationships with clinical directors, hospital consultants, general practitioners and health organisations. He provides expert, innovative and proactive advice and is a key contributor in shaping the overall strategy, decision making and medical vision within his trust.

Professor Pickuth has extensive expertise in service transformation, in strengthening the strategic positioning of a trust and in service improvement. Combining a systemic holistic manner, excellence in his speciality and strong business acumen, he is a charismatic leader in how to effectively translate strategic business decisions into operational project management. He offers a specialist background in harmonising medical responsibility to meet economic targets, promote strategic alliances and shape organisational visions – including developing strategy concepts across traditional boundaries and care systems.

Please email the author at **healthcareexecutives@yahoo.com**

FOREWORD

As Professor of Radiology at the Royal Marsden Hospital and the Institute of Cancer Research, London, for over 30 years I have witnessed some of the most extraordinary advances in the history of medicine. These include the birth of the technological revolution in diagnostic imaging, led by the introduction of CT and MRI, the successful innovation and development of new drug programmes which have resulted in improved outcomes for patients, and the continued advance of surgical techniques which have also had a huge positive impact on patient survival rates.

Equally important over these decades has been the recognition of the need for robust systems to manage healthcare within a strategic and operational framework to provide the best care for patients in the most cost effective way. While much progress has clearly been made in all these areas, the challenges faced by healthcare services to provide the very best care for every single patient on every single day are relentless, and continue to grow.

Successful modern healthcare systems are those which are patient focused, cost effective and continuously improving. In order to achieve these objectives, it is imperative that clinicians and managers work together seamlessly to provide an integrated approach with common goals and within a culture of trust, shared experience and learning. This requires strong leadership and commitment from both clinicians and managers at every level throughout an organisation.

As Medical Director during the latter years of my career, I learnt an enormous amount about successful leadership and management by working closely with the Chief Executive Officer of the Royal Marsden Hospital, Miss Cally Palmer, CBE, and her entire team. This new world of increasing regulation and of balancing high quality clinical performance and continuous improvement with service efficiency and meeting very ambitious financial targets was crucially important to the success of the Royal Marsden Hospital as one of the first wave Foundation Trusts within the National Health Service (NHS). Cally inspired my further interest in healthcare management in my future roles as President of the British Institute of Radiology, President of the Royal College of Radiologists and, more recently, as a Non-Executive Director both at the Royal Marsden Hospital and within the independent sector.

Professor Dirk Pickuth, Medical Director of the Caritas Hospital Foundation Trust and Head of the Department of Radiology at the Caritas Academic Teaching Hospital in Saarbrücken, Germany, has compiled his vast knowledge and expertise in medical leadership and management to give the reader a wonderful tapestry of best practice guidance. Dirk draws on his personal experience in very senior managerial roles as well as his highly regarded clinical and academic reputation as a leading figure in international radiology.

Dirk undertook a Clinical Research Fellowship in Radiology in our department at the Royal Marsden Hospital from 1991 to 1992. It was during this Fellowship that he stood out as an exceptional young doctor with extraordinary commitment and incredible enthusiasm for achieving excellence in each and every aspect of his clinical and academic work. Dirk attained and sustained peak performance at all times, was always a role model for other colleagues and put collective needs before his own needs. His positive energy and inspirational demeanour encouraged and empowered those around him to reach their full potential.

We established a long-term friendship, and over the years I have been fortunate to witness Dirk's enormous success as his career has continued to broaden and flourish into the leading role in healthcare that he enjoys today. Over the years, Dirk has gained a deep understanding of the history, development and framework of healthcare systems in several countries, with a strong interest in the NHS as well as the governance systems embedded within its matrix. He is a highly acclaimed and truly exceptional leader and manager, innovator and reformer.

Dirk has brought all his vast experience together in this exciting and informative book on leadership and management in healthcare. Enhancing management priorities, developing robust hospital strategies, business planning, promoting effective communication techniques and resolving challenging issues are among the many topics covered in this very readable and highly systematic text. This book will therefore appeal to a wide audience of healthcare leaders, managers and clinicians across international boundaries, but will have particular relevance to those interested in the complex organisational structures in Britain, as Dirk focuses on the framework of the NHS to provide the reader with much valuable information on its organisational structure and code of practice.

A major attraction of this book is the succinct and clear format of the text, with fact boxes, bullet points, expert insights and practical tips. Suggestions for further reading add a useful dimension for those wishing to explore particular topics in more detail.

I know that if I had been able to have this little gem during my time as a medical leader, it would have been close to hand for quick reference at all times and would have helped me resolve the various issues and scenarios that healthcare leaders deal with in everyday practice. The book also provides useful information on how to manage more complex challenges, such as coping with poor performance within a team or on an individual basis and dealing with bullying and harassment. Other useful chapters cover appraisal and revalidation of doctors as well as the role of the various professional bodies in underpinning high quality care.

Dirk is wholeheartedly Anglophile. The supplementary chapters on Britain are entertaining and fun to read, giving a snapshot of Britishness, and, although I was born and bred in England, there were several little aspects of our culture of which I was totally unaware until I read this wonderful book.

This text is indeed a 'must get' for all aspiring managers and medically qualified individuals who are interested in developing their management skills. It will also be the perfect tool for experienced leaders as an aide-mémoire and to provide a check list for thorough preparation of various activities and for resolving problems.

I recommend this book to you all most highly as an inspirational and compelling read.

Professor Dame Janet Husband DBE, FMedSci, FRCP, FRCR
Emeritus Professor of Radiology
The Royal Marsden Hospital and The Institute of Cancer Research
London, United Kingdom

PREFACE

The aim of this book is to inform and inspire you, while challenging and encouraging you in your leadership and management role.

Healthcare executives create ideas, deliver messages and provide context while radiating confidence, conveying trust and leveraging energy. They are dedicated, enthusiastic and passionate professionals who embody purpose, vision and strategy. They never walk alone; they have their team, they empower other people. They aspire and inspire.

Great leaders are successful.

Extraordinary leaders make extraordinary things happen.

Outstanding leaders are humble.

Healthcare leadership and management, however, is not an area for the faint of heart. Healthcare executives are required to make difficult decisions under significant scrutiny from politicians, the media and the public.

This book is designed to provide healthcare professionals with the knowledge they need for leadership positions. It addresses structures, topics and issues while providing an actionable framework for developing and applying leadership skills.

Each chapter, subchapter and factbox in the book is self-contained.

Starting with an initial overview – from a healthcare perspective – of trends, globalisation, systems and rankings, the book then proceeds to explain healthcare structure, constitution, values and ethics. This complex material has been deliberately presented in a concise manner for a speedy read by busy individuals. Key chapters cover legislation, resources, finance and commissioning. Additional chapters are dedicated to healthcare services and infrastructure. This systematic overview helps you make sense of and navigate through the changing waters of modern healthcare while imparting fundamental knowledge of business administration.

It is essential that leaders at any level clearly understand topics such as regulation, inspection, reviews and governance. A breakdown of these themes explains essential facts and key issues to allow easier comprehension for any professional, whatever their background. Organisations and bodies, remits and responsibilities are described. Healthcare risks are discussed in a separate chapter.

Safety, quality and audit are fundamental in achieving high standards in modern healthcare. These subjects are covered using a structured and disciplined approach with the help of checklists and templates. Chapters cover practical details: incidents, safeguarding and complaints, and how to handle them.

Whistleblowing, concerns and litigation play an increasing role in healthcare. It is vital that executives possess a basic knowledge of these core issues, which are covered in consecutive chapters.

Healthcare information management and information technology are outlined in subsequent chapters.

The following units contain factsheets on healthcare challenges, transformation and personalisation. To help you quickly absorb and apply the information, the chapters concentrate on typical scenarios and trusted solutions.

Special attention is given to all aspects surrounding work in the field of healthcare. Chapter topics include jobs, employment and diversity. This material serves as a comprehensive source of easy-to-use materials for staff management.

A leader's most important job is communication, a vital area which constitutes a large part of this book. Reflecting on recent evidence, the most efficient communication techniques in the modern healthcare environment are presented, ideas you can immediately put into practice to lead and effect change within your organisation.

Issues that are faced daily by healthcare executives are also covered in subsequent chapters. Key themes of leadership and management activities include meetings, presentations, negotiations and projects. These topics are relevant to both emerging and established executives, and the book covers up-to-date information and on-the-spot guidance to help in mastering day-to-day issues. Concise insights provide realistic ideas and thoughtful advice to help you reach your full potential and make a real difference.

Special chapters are devoted to workflow, performance and productivity issues, focusing on both individual and organisational assessment and development. This material provides easy-to-apply strategies for engaging and improving leadership and management. Critical aspects of appraisal are also covered.

The chapters covering talents, teams and the personalities and skillsets of managers and leaders are a valuable resource for new managers and seasoned leaders alike. The lessons contained here feature personal experiences, wisdom, insights and principles that will help you reach the top and stay there. The toolkits give you modern concepts and best practices at your fingertips.

The next theme focuses on healthcare executives, with an emphasis on Board Chairs, Chief Executives and Medical Directors. Recruitment, roles, qualifications and responsibilities are presented in subchapters. These sections also contain numerous practical tips for healthcare executives.

The final chapter is dedicated to outstanding leaders from around the world. Outstanding leaders are people who have shifted from success to significance. These cream-of-the-crop individuals serve as role models at all levels and in all situations – and they create a culture of excellence in healthcare.

The supplementary chapters are aimed at international residents working and living in the United Kingdom. The material provides information on the country, its history and its language. These lists are arranged in chronological or geographical order and then alphabetically or by preference. The book concludes with business phrases and essential grammar for executives whose first language is not English.

All facts are from reference sources which are listed in the bibliography at the end of this book. I will be happy to correct any inaccuracies in later editions.

Over the past quarter of a century, I have had the privilege of studying, working and teaching in several countries around the globe. I have engaged with many distinguished executives and clinicians from public and private healthcare organisations. It has been a tremendous honour to have met inspiring global leaders during my work in establishing exchange programmes and cooperation projects.

Written in a personal capacity, this book reflects my hands-on experience as Medical Director and Department Head in various healthcare settings. It is designed for practitioners, by a practitioner.

Since time is scarce and precious for all of us, I have favoured a note format wherever possible. The text boxes represent individual facts, are free-standing and provide clear structure, enabling you to open the book at any section and begin reading in whatever timeframe suits you. The tips are tried and tested and are intended to inspire you, even while you are on the move.

I sincerely hope that you enjoy this book and find it relevant, useful and rewarding.

Professor Dirk Pickuth MD, PhD, MDs (honoris causa)

ACKNOWLEDGEMENTS

Our patients are at the heart of our care – hats off to the dedicated, hardworking and compassionate women and men in healthcare around the world.

From a young age I was surrounded by inspiring, strong and powerful professors, both in London and in Edinburgh, and each of these personalities encouraged me to achieve my potential. I could not have wished for better support and insight from such an outstanding group of academics.

I wish to offer my sincere thanks to all who contributed to this publication, in particular to the many colleagues and friends in the United Kingdom who took the time and trouble to read and comment on numerous topics and chapters of the book.

Many thanks to Silke Dauber, my executive assistant, for her tireless support and great enthusiasm.

I was fortunate to have the services of a first-class editor and proofreader, Helen Stevens, of Saltaire Editorial Services. My warmest thanks to her for suggestions above and beyond the call of duty.

I am very grateful to Sandra Board, of Sanded Script Editing & Proofreading, and Moira Hunter, of wordforword design, who proofread the manuscript from front to back.

Special thanks to Jem Butcher, of Jem Butcher Design, for his truly amazing creativity and the superb cover design.

I extend my greatest thanks to Bill Baty, David Joyce and Adam Wilkinson, of Tech-Set Ltd, for designing and typesetting the book. It has been an incredible pleasure to work with this brilliant team.

I would also like to acknowledge the exceptionally professional team at Troubador Publishing Ltd for their advice, efficiency and kindness.

Lastly, I express my heartfelt appreciation to my family and friends for their support and encouragement in this overwhelming undertaking.

Professor Dirk Pickuth MD, PhD, MDs (honoris causa)

1 HEALTHCARE TRENDS

CHAPTER OVERVIEW

▶ **TRENDS IN HEALTHCARE**

TRENDS IN HEALTHCARE

▶ Medicine moves from a care approach towards a health approach.
▶ Medicine moves from hospital to home.
  • Preventing an illness becomes more important than treating an illness.
▶ Medicine moves from a reactive approach towards a proactive approach.

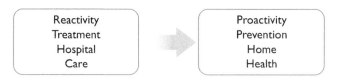

▶ Medicine evolves from occasional hospital-based care towards permanent patient-centred concepts.

▶ Medical knowledge increases at record speed.

▶ Medicine becomes multidisciplinary, guidelines oriented, evidence based and standardised.

▶ Standardisation in medicine
- Reducing complexity
- Reducing variation
- Improving cooperation
- Improving communication
- Enhancing safety
- Enhancing quality

▶ Patients at the heart of healthcare
▶ Technology at the heart of progress
- Big data
- Artificial intelligence
- Functional genomics
- Precision medicine
▶ IT at the heart of implementation

▶ Patients are remotely connected to the healthcare system.

2 HEALTHCARE GLOBALISATION

CHAPTER OVERVIEW

▶ **GLOBALISATION OF HEALTHCARE**

GLOBALISATION OF HEALTHCARE

▶ Medicine is international and thrives on the interchange of knowledge and experience.

▶ Different countries – The same daily problems.
▶ All countries and all systems have something to learn and something to teach.
▶ What works – What does not work.

| Learning from each other | Sharing ideas and possibilities | Encouraging adaptation and adoption | Benefiting from each other |

▶ Global knowledge and expertise transfer
  • Exchanging policies
    ▪ Example: Cost effectiveness studies
  • Standardising and harmonising care
    ▪ Example: Evidence based medicine
  • Enhancing quality
    ▪ Example: International specialist opinion

▶ Today's healthcare executives should have extensive international experience.

3 HEALTHCARE SYSTEMS

CHAPTER OVERVIEW

- ▶ EVOLUTION OF HEALTHCARE SYSTEMS
- ▶ DEVELOPMENT OF HEALTHCARE SYSTEMS
- ▶ AIMS OF HEALTHCARE SYSTEMS
- ▶ PROBLEMS OF HEALTHCARE SYSTEMS
- ▶ APPROACHES TO HEALTHCARE SYSTEMS

EVOLUTION OF HEALTHCARE SYSTEMS

- ▶ Complex result of several factors
  - History
  - Culture
  - Politics
  - Economy
  - Science
  - Teaching

DEVELOPMENT OF HEALTHCARE SYSTEMS

- ▶ Complex product of several factors
  - Political challenges
  - Economic challenges
  - Social challenges
  - Ethical challenges
  - Technical challenges
  - Situational challenges

AIMS OF HEALTHCARE SYSTEMS

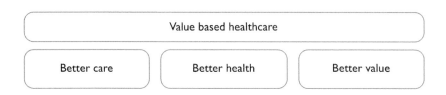

Value based healthcare		
Better care	Better health	Better value

▶ Value based healthcare: Patient health outcomes (numerator) relative to the total cost of resources used to deliver these outcomes (denominator)
  ● Defined for a specific medical condition over the full care cycle

▶ Personal value: Value for the patient
▶ Procedural value: Value for the intervention
▶ Allocative value: Value for the public

PROBLEMS OF HEALTHCARE SYSTEMS

▶ Ageing population
▶ Public expectations
▶ Rising demand
▶ Funding gaps
▶ Staff shortages
▶ Quality issues

▶ Inequality
▶ Duplication
▶ Fragmentation
▶ Variation

▶ The 'VUCA' world
  ● Volatility
  ● Uncertainty
  ● Complexity
  ● Ambiguity

▶ Healthcare systems always need to keep pace.
  • The time to act is always now.
▶ Healthcare systems always need to be sustainable.

▶ Often a broad consensus on reforms
▶ Rarely a clear path for reforms

▶ Lack of both capacity and capability of leadership

APPROACHES TO HEALTHCARE SYSTEMS

▶ Social solidarity
▶ Individual responsibility

▶ Strong vision
▶ Patient focus
  • Safe, effective, efficient, equitable
▶ Care integration
▶ Supportive environment
  • Political, financial, legal, educational

▶ Developing leaders
▶ Empowering staff
▶ Mobilising communities
▶ Engaging patients
▶ Innovating care
▶ Exploiting technology
▶ Optimising processes
▶ Reducing bureaucracy
▶ Streamlining procurement
▶ Controlling costs
▶ Driving efficiency
▶ Creating value

4 HEALTHCARE RANKINGS

CHAPTER OVERVIEW

▶ SELECTED COUNTRIES WITH BEST PRACTICE
▶ COUNTRY RANKINGS ON HEALTHCARE PERFORMANCE
▶ UNITED KINGDOM AND HEALTHCARE PERFORMANCE

SELECTED COUNTRIES WITH BEST PRACTICE

▶ Australia: Mental care
▶ Brazil: Community care
▶ India: Creative care
▶ Israel: Primary care
▶ Japan: Elderly care
▶ Scandinavia: Prevention
▶ Singapore: IT
▶ Switzerland: Funding
▶ UK: Universality
▶ USA: Research

COUNTRY RANKINGS ON HEALTHCARE PERFORMANCE

▶ Most rankings without meaningful criteria and substantial methodology
▶ First places in ranking attempts, in alphabetical order
  • Japan
  • Scandinavia
  • Singapore
  • Switzerland
  • UK

UNITED KINGDOM AND HEALTHCARE PERFORMANCE

▶ 2013: Ranked the highest performing health system of eleven industrialised countries by the Commonwealth Fund
  - Number one in quality care
    ▪ Effective care
    ▪ Safe care
    ▪ Co-ordinated care
    ▪ Patient-centred care
  - Number one in access
  - Number one in efficient care
  - Number one in values
▶ 2017: Ranked the highest performing health system of eleven industrialised countries by the Commonwealth Fund
  - Number one in care process
  - Number one in healthcare equity

▶ The NHS is the highest performing healthcare system, although it is underfunded compared to other countries.

▶ The NHS is universal, value based and equitable.

National Health Service		
Universal	Value based	Equitable

▶ The NHS has the advantage of a substantial relationship between clinical practice, scientific research and academic teaching.

National Health Service		
Clinical practice	Scientific research	Academic teaching

5 HEALTHCARE STRUCTURE

CHAPTER OVERVIEW

▶ HISTORY OF THE NHS
▶ THE HEALTH AND SOCIAL CARE ACT 2012
▶ THE NEW NHS ENGLAND 2013
▶ STRUCTURE OF THE NHS
▶ PARLIAMENT
▶ DEPARTMENT OF HEALTH
▶ COMMISSIONING
▶ HEALTHCARE SERVICES
▶ MONITORING AND REGULATION
▶ DATA AND EVIDENCE
▶ TRAINING AND DEVELOPMENT
▶ THE NHS IN THE OTHER THREE COUNTRIES OF THE UK
▶ INDEPENDENT PROVIDERS

HISTORY OF THE NHS

▶ Foundation
- 5th July 1948
- Labour Government
- Aneurin 'Nye' Bevan
▶ Principles
- Publicly funded system
- Based on clinical need and not ability to pay, free at the point of use
- Available to all

▶ 'The essence of a satisfactory health service is that the rich and the poor are treated alike.' (Aneurin Bevan)

▶ The NHS is the greatest achievement of social democracy in Britain.

THE HEALTH AND SOCIAL CARE ACT 2012

▶ Clinically led commissioning
  • Previously: Primary Care Trusts
  • Now: Clinical Commissioning Groups
    ▪ Commissioning as a process through which the health needs of the local population are identified and the health services purchased to meet those needs
▶ Increased patient involvement
  • Local consumer champion organisation: Local Healthwatch
  • National consumer champion organisation: Healthwatch England
▶ Public health focus
  • Public Health England
▶ Streamlined arm's-length bodies
▶ Healthcare market competition
  • Independent providers
    ▪ Private companies
    ▪ Voluntary organisations
    ▪ Social enterprises

THE NEW NHS ENGLAND 2013

▶ New structure
▶ New organisations and bodies
▶ New remits and responsibilities
▶ New opportunities

STRUCTURE OF THE NHS

Political level	Parliament
Strategic level	Department of Health
Operational level	Commissioning
	Healthcare services
	Monitoring and regulation
	Data and evidence
	Training and development

PARLIAMENT

▶ Exercises political oversight of public health, the NHS and social care
▶ Scrutinises through political debates, MPs' questions to ministers and select committees

▶ Select committees
- Consider policy issues
- Scrutinise the government's work and spending
- Examine legislation proposals

▶ Select committees particularly relevant to NHS England
- Health and Social Care Committee
- Public Accounts Committee
- Housing, Communities and Local Government Committee
- Public Administration and Constitutional Affairs Committee

DEPARTMENT OF HEALTH

▶ Official name: Department of Health and Social Care

▶ Secretary of State for Health
- Is an important member of the cabinet
- Retains an overarching duty for the NHS
- Has the overall responsibility for strategic leadership
- Produces an annual report for the parliament

- ▶ Minister of State for Health
- ▶ Parliamentary Under Secretary of State for Health

- ▶ Strategic leadership for public health, the NHS and social care
  - Sets policy
  - Maintains legislation
  - Defines outcomes
  - Provides leadership
  - Manages relationships
  - Secures resources
- ▶ Strategic responsibility for arm's-length bodies
  - Public Health England
  - Care Quality Commission
  - Health Education England
  - National Institute for Health and Care Excellence
  - NHS Improvement
  - NHS Digital
  - NHS Resolution

COMMISSIONING

- ▶ NHS England
- ▶ Public Health England
- ▶ Health and Wellbeing Boards
  - Local authorities
  - Clinical commissioning groups
  - Local Healthwatch

HEALTHCARE SERVICES

- ▶ Locally commissioned services
  - Secondary care
    - Hospital care, treatment centres
  - Community services
    - Allied health professionals, community nursing services, health visitors, community midwives

- Local public health services
- Mental health
- Rehabilitation services
▶ Nationally commissioned services
  - Primary care
    - Medical, dental, pharmacy and optical services
  - Specialised healthcare
    - Low-volume, high-cost, centralised and specialised services
  - Immunisation, children, screening, prevention
  - Military healthcare
  - Offender healthcare

MONITORING AND REGULATION

▶ Care Quality Commission
▶ NHS Improvement
▶ Healthwatch

DATA AND EVIDENCE

▶ National Institute for Health and Care Excellence
▶ NHS Digital

TRAINING AND DEVELOPMENT

▶ Health Education England
▶ Local Education and Training Boards
▶ Local education providers

THE NHS IN THE OTHER THREE COUNTRIES OF THE UK

	Political oversight of the NHS	Strategic leadership of the NHS
Scotland	Scottish Parliament	Scottish Government Health and Social Care Directorate
Wales	National Assembly for Wales	Welsh Department of Health and Social Services
Northern Ireland	Northern Ireland Assembly	Northern Ireland's Department of Health

INDEPENDENT PROVIDERS

- ▶ 'Any qualified provider'
- ▶ How to qualify
  - • Being licensed
  - • Being registered
  - • Meeting the terms and conditions of the NHS standard contract
    - ▪ Abiding by the NHS Constitution, relevant guidance and the law
  - • Accepting NHS prices
  - • Meeting service requirements

6 HEALTHCARE CONSTITUTION

CHAPTER OVERVIEW

► **NHS CONSTITUTION**
► **PRINCIPLES**
► **VALUES**
► **RIGHTS**
► **PLEDGES**
► **RESPONSIBILITIES**

NHS CONSTITUTION

► Specifies what patients, staff and the public can expect from the NHS
► Specifies what the NHS expects from patients, staff and the public in return

► Cannot be altered by the government without the involvement of patients, staff and the public
► Will be renewed every ten years
  • Handbook to the Constitution to be renewed at least every three years

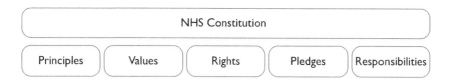

PRINCIPLES

► The NHS provides a comprehensive service, available to all.
► Access to NHS services is based on clinical need, not an individual's ability to pay.

- ▶ The NHS aspires to the highest standards of excellence and professionalism.
- ▶ The NHS aspires to put patients at the heart of everything it does.
- ▶ The NHS works across organisational boundaries and in partnership with other organisations in the interest of patients, local communities and the wider population.
- ▶ The NHS is committed to providing best value for taxpayers' money and the most effective, fair and sustainable use of finite resources.
- ▶ The NHS is accountable to the public, communities and patients that it serves.

VALUES

- ▶ Working together for patients
- ▶ Respect and dignity
- ▶ Commitment to quality of care
- ▶ Compassion
- ▶ Improving lives
- ▶ Everyone counts

RIGHTS

- ▶ Access to health services
- ▶ Quality of care and environment
- ▶ Nationally approved treatments, drugs and programmes
- ▶ Respect, consent and confidentiality
- ▶ Informed choice
- ▶ Involvement in personal healthcare and in the NHS
- ▶ Complaint and redress

PLEDGES

- ▶ Pledges as a commitment by the NHS to provide
  - Comprehensive high quality services
  - High quality working environments
    - ▪ Pledges not legally binding

RESPONSIBILITIES

- ▶ Things people can do for themselves and for one another to help the NHS work effectively, and to ensure resources are used responsibly

7 HEALTHCARE VALUES

CHAPTER OVERVIEW

▶ HEALTHCARE VALUES
▶ NHS VALUES

HEALTHCARE VALUES

Treating all people with dignity, compassion and respect

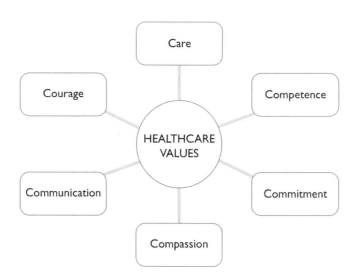

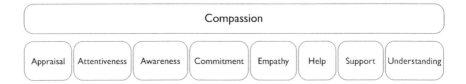

NHS VALUES

▶ Describe core aspirations of NHS services
- Derive from discussions with patients, staff and the public

▶ Facilitate collaborative working at all levels

▶ Patients come first
▶ Improvement of health
▶ Commitment to quality
- Safety, patient experience, effectiveness

▶ Care with compassion
▶ Respect and dignity
▶ Everybody is included

8 HEALTHCARE ETHICS

CHAPTER OVERVIEW

▶ PRINCIPLISM
▶ BIOETHICS
▶ RATIONING

PRINCIPLISM

▶ System of ethics
- Most widely recognised and universally adopted bioethical theory
- Compatible with most intellectual, cultural and religious beliefs

▶ Four moral principles

Principlism			
Autonomy	Beneficence	Nonmalfeasance	Justice

▶ Autonomy
- Free will
▶ Beneficence
- Only good
▶ Nonmalfeasance
- No harm
▶ Justice
- Social distribution

BIOETHICS

▶ Medical decision making
- From the protection and paternalism-based model ('doctor knows best')
- To the enablement and autonomy-based model ('competent adult patient')

RATIONING

▶ Waiting lists
▶ 'Postcode lottery'
- Decisions taken at local level about which services and treatments can or cannot be provided

▶ Fair allocation in view of scarce resources
- First step: National Institute for Health and Care Excellence
  - Does the cost effectiveness of the treatment justify NHS provision?
- Second step: If denied treatment, application for exceptional case funding
- Third step: If denied funding, judicial review

9 HEALTHCARE LEGISLATION

CHAPTER OVERVIEW

- ► DISCLAIMER
- ► CAPACITY
- ► CONFIDENTIALITY
- ► CONSENT
- ► NEGLIGENCE
- ► MANSLAUGHTER
- ► RESEARCH

DISCLAIMER

► The factsheets in this book are not intended as legal advice. Consult an expert on the specifics of your issue.

CAPACITY

- ► Mental Capacity Act
  - Patient has capacity
    - Unless proven otherwise
    - To decide for himself/herself whether to be treated
  - Patient lacks capacity
    - Test for capacity
    - To be treated according to his/her best interest

- ► Lack of capacity
  - Temporary or permanent impairment or disturbance of the mind or brain
    - Unable to understand the information
    - Unable to retain the information

21

- Unable to weigh the information
- Unable to communicate a decision

▶ A patient does not lack capacity simply because he/she makes an unwise decision.

▶ Capacity must be reached without undue influence or coercion.

▶ An adult competent patient can refuse medical treatment.
▶ An adult competent patient can refuse lifesaving treatment.
  - Where there is doubt, the sanctity of life prevails and the refusal of the patient will be overridden.

▶ Mental Capacity Act
  - An act done or decision made must be in the incompetent patient's best interest.

▶ Mental Capacity Act
  - Patient to participate in the decision making process as far as possible
  - Patient's past and present wishes, beliefs and values to be taken into account
  - LPA, Deputy and anyone interested in the patient's welfare to be consulted

▶ Mental Capacity Act
  - The act must be conducted in the least restrictive way.

CONFIDENTIALITY

▶ Equitable common law duty

▶ Exceptions to the duty of confidentiality
  - Express consent
  - Implied consent
  - Public interest
  - Statutory provisions

CONSENT

▶ A patient's consent is the cornerstone of lawful treatment.

▶ Failure to inform the patient in broad terms about the treatment could lead to an action in negligence or an action in battery.

▶ How much information does a patient need in order to be properly or adequately informed? Doctors should provide whatever information matters to the individual patient. Reasonable doctors follow professional guidelines.

▶ Consent and lack of capacity
  - Lasting Power of Attorney
  - Advance decisions
    ▪ Right of self-determination and of autonomy
  - Court of Protection Deputy

▶ Consent and a child between the ages of 16 and 18
  - There is a rebuttable presumption that this child can consent to medical treatment.
    ▪ No reference to any ability to refuse treatment

▶ Consent and a child under the age of 16
  - This child can consent to medical treatment if he/she is considered Gillick competent; that is, he/she must be sufficiently mature to appreciate the medical advice.

NEGLIGENCE

▶ Elements of negligence
  - Duty of care
  - Breach of duty
  - Causation
  - Harm

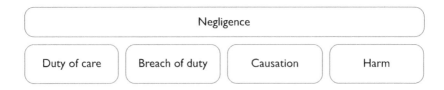

Negligence			
Duty of care	Breach of duty	Causation	Harm

▶ According to the Bolam test, as modified by Bolitho, a doctor is not guilty of negligence if he/she has acted in accordance with a practice accepted as proper by a responsible body of medical opinion, provided that this opinion is capable of withstanding logical analysis.

MANSLAUGHTER

▶ Corporate Manslaughter Act
  • Gross failures in the management of health and safety with fatal consequences

RESEARCH

▶ Health Research Authority
  • National system for the governance of health research
    ▪ Promoting transparency in research
    ▪ Making sure research is ethically reviewed and approved
    ▪ Overseeing committees and services

▶ All clinical trials must, in the first place, be approved by a research ethics committee.

▶ Consent of patients for participation in research must be informed as well as voluntary.

▶ The Health Research Authority provides independent recommendations on the processing of identifiable patient information where it is not always practical to obtain consent, for research and non-research projects.

10 HEALTHCARE RESOURCES

CHAPTER OVERVIEW

▶ **RESOURCE TYPES**
▶ **FINANCIAL RESOURCES**
▶ **HUMAN RESOURCES**
▶ **VALUE BASED RECRUITMENT**
▶ **SOCIAL CARE COMMITMENT**
▶ **INFRASTRUCTURAL RESOURCES**
▶ **EMOTIONAL RESOURCES**
▶ **RESOURCE MANAGEMENT**

RESOURCE TYPES

▶ Financial resources
▶ Human resources
▶ Infrastructural resources
▶ Emotional resources

FINANCIAL RESOURCES

▶ Number of people paying for health services
▶ Amount of money these people are paying

HUMAN RESOURCES

▶ Value based recruitment
▶ Social care commitment

VALUE BASED RECRUITMENT

▶ Identifying workplace values
▶ Embedding workplace values
▶ Checking workplace values
▶ Recruitment, selection, retention
▶ Information, induction, support
▶ Supervision, appraisal, progression

SOCIAL CARE COMMITMENT

▶ Selecting workforce
▶ Providing induction
▶ Strengthening skills
▶ Upholding standards
▶ Taking responsibility
▶ Supervising employees
▶ Supporting staff

INFRASTRUCTURAL RESOURCES

▶ Estates
▶ Buildings
▶ Facilities
▶ Amenities
▶ Supplies
▶ IT

EMOTIONAL RESOURCES

▶ Commitment
▶ 'Going the extra mile'
▶ Compassion

RESOURCE MANAGEMENT

▶ Workforce allocation in relation to resource management

▶ Voluntary support in relation to an inclusive vision

▶ Patient satisfaction in relation to health outcomes

▶ The right amount of the right resource needs to be in the right place at the right time.

▶ The right people need to be valued every day and every minute and every second.

11 HEALTHCARE FINANCE

CHAPTER OVERVIEW

- ► HEALTHCARE FINANCE
- ► NHS FINANCE
- ► ARM'S-LENGTH BODY
- ► NHS BUDGET
- ► CCG BUDGET
- ► PROVIDER BUDGET
- ► KEY ORGANISATIONS
- ► REVENUE CYCLE
- ► FINANCIAL STATEMENT
- ► FINANCIAL RATIOS
- ► FINANCIAL PERFORMANCE
- ► ANNUAL BUDGET
- ► VARIANCE ANALYSIS
- ► STRATEGIC PLANNING
- ► BUSINESS PLANNING
- ► BUSINESS INTELLIGENCE
- ► HEALTH ECONOMICS

HEALTHCARE FINANCE

► Healthcare executives need to be commercially focused and financially literate because money is the ultimate measure of the sustainable success of all organisations.

NHS FINANCE

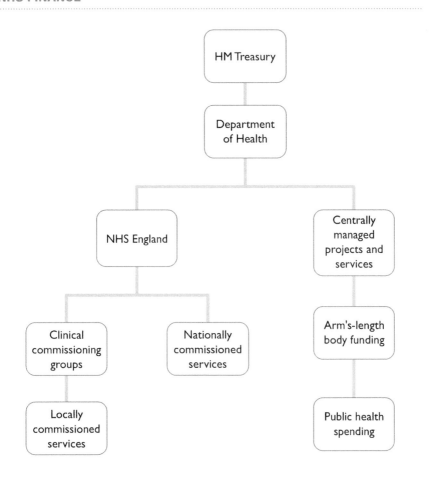

ARM'S-LENGTH BODY

▶ An organisation that delivers a public service, that is not a ministerial government department and that operates to a greater or lesser extent at a distance from ministers

▶ Functions for the NHS
  - Regulating the healthcare system and workforce
  - Establishing standards
  - Protecting patients
  - Providing central services to the NHS

29

NHS BUDGET

- ▶ Funding sources
  - Taxes
  - National Insurance contributions
  - Charges
    - Prescriptions
    - Dental services
    - Glasses
- ▶ Resource allocation
  - Spending review of HM Treasury
    - Every two to three years

CCG BUDGET

- ▶ Weighted capitation basis
  - Based on
    - Size of the population
  - Adjusted for
    - Health of the population
    - Age profile of the population
    - Location of the population

PROVIDER BUDGET

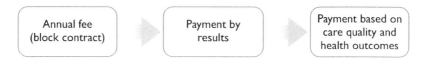

Annual fee (block contract) → Payment by results → Payment based on care quality and health outcomes

KEY ORGANISATIONS

- ▶ NHS Shared Business Services
  - Finance, accounting, human resources, payroll, procurement
- ▶ NHS Business Services Authority
  - Payment, reimbursement, remuneration and reconciliation for patients and employees
  - NHS pension scheme

▶ NHS Supply Chain
  ● Procurement, logistics, e-commerce, customer support, supplier support
▶ NHS Counter Fraud Authority
  ● Protection of resources from fraud

REVENUE CYCLE

▶ Complete medical billing process from beginning to end

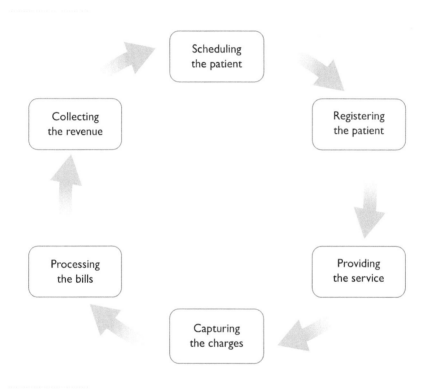

▶ Making or breaking the success of an organisation
  ● Accurate documentation
  ● Accurate coding
  ● Accurate billing
  ● Accurate control

FINANCIAL STATEMENT

▶ Formal record of the financial activities and the business position

▶ Balance sheet
  ● Assets, liabilities, equity
▶ Income statement
  ● Revenues, expenses, gains, losses
▶ Cash flow
  ● Operating, investing, financing

FINANCIAL RATIOS

▶ Analysis of the financial health of an organisation
  ● Comparison against previous periods
  ● Comparison against other organisations
  ● Comparison against targets
  ● Comparison against benchmarks

▶ Profitability ratios
▶ Liquidity ratios
▶ Debt ratios
▶ Asset ratios

FINANCIAL PERFORMANCE

▶ Sustainability
  ● Capital service cover
  ● Liquidity
▶ Efficiency
  ● Income and expenditure margin
▶ Controls
  ● Performance against plan

ANNUAL BUDGET

▶ Spending plan
- Productivity
- Revenues
- Expenses
  - Evaluating the business
  - Reviewing the potential
  - Allocating the resources
  - Controlling the performance
  - Developing the business

VARIANCE ANALYSIS

▶ Analysis of actual results versus budgeted results
- Providing an early indication of negative variations
- Highlighting developing trends and necessary interventions
- Adjusting the financial strategies and business operations

STRATEGIC PLANNING

▶ Analysing situations
▶ Setting goals
▶ Determining actions
▶ Allocating resources
- SWOT analysis
  - Strengths, weaknesses, opportunities, threats
- PESTLE analysis
  - Political, economic, social, technological, legal, environmental
- Scenario planning
- Balanced scorecard

BUSINESS PLANNING

▶ Statement of business goals and plan for achieving goals
  - Executive summary
  - Vision statement
  - Organisation description
  - Organisation analysis
  - Competitor analysis
  - Market analysis
  - Marketing plan
  - Operations plan
  - Management plan
  - Financial plan

BUSINESS INTELLIGENCE

▶ Benchmarking is comparing the structure, processes and performance of one healthcare organisation with its peer organisations.

▶ Best practice is a method which consistently shows results achieved by one means to be superior to those achieved by other means.

▶ Key performance indicators are measurable values which demonstrate how effectively a healthcare organisation is achieving key business objectives.

▶ Dashboards are visual displays of important information tailored to the specific requirements and consolidated into a single screen.

▶ Key features of quality dashboards
  - Immediacy
  - Intuitiveness
  - Simplicity

▶ Performance measurement and documentation
  - Reports
  - Benchmarks
  - Critical success factors
  - Key performance indicators
  - Patient satisfaction metrics
  - Performance dashboards
  - Balanced scorecard

HEALTH ECONOMICS

▶ Health economics offers a systematic approach to decision making in healthcare. It helps in the management of issues of choice and scarcity.

▶ Key questions
  - How do we get the greatest good for the greatest number?
  - How do we get the greatest outcome from the available resources?

▶ Economic considerations
  - What does the system want to achieve?
  - What are the different options for achieving this?
  - How do these options compare with each other?
  - What costs are involved for each option?

▶ Economic evaluation
  - Cost minimisation analysis
  - Cost effectiveness analysis
  - Cost utility analysis
  - Cost benefit analysis

12 HEALTHCARE COMMISSIONING

CHAPTER OVERVIEW

► **NHS FUNCTIONS**
► **COMMISSIONING DEFINITION**
► **COMMISSIONING PROCESS**
► **DESIGN OF CLINICAL COMMISSIONING GROUPS**
► **GOVERNANCE OF CLINICAL COMMISSIONING GROUPS**
► **SERVICES OF CLINICAL COMMISSIONING GROUPS**
► **SUPPORT FOR CLINICAL COMMISSIONING GROUPS**
► **COMMISSIONING TRENDS**
► **RIGHT OF CHOICE**
► **PATIENT CHOICE AND COMPLAINTS SYSTEM**
► **HEALTH AND WELLBEING BOARDS**

NHS FUNCTIONS

► Functions of the day-to-day operations of the NHS
  - Commissioning services
  - Providing services
► Functions of NHS England in particular
  - National leadership for care quality and health outcomes
  - Overseeing the operation of clinical commissioning groups
  - Allocating resources to clinical commissioning groups
  - Nationally commissioned services
    - Primary care
    - Specialised healthcare
    - Immunisation, children, screening, prevention
    - Military healthcare
    - Offender healthcare

▶ Discharge of NHS England's responsibilities
  ● 1 national team
  ● 5 regional teams
    ▪ London
    ▪ North
    ▪ Midlands and East
    ▪ South East
    ▪ South West
  ● 27 area teams
▶ Mandate of NHS England's duties
  ● Published yearly
  ● Objectives for the NHS and its budget
  ● Political control
    ▪ NHS accountable to the parliament
    ▪ NHS accountable to the public

COMMISSIONING DEFINITION

▶ Process by which services are planned and provided to meet the population's needs

COMMISSIONING PROCESS

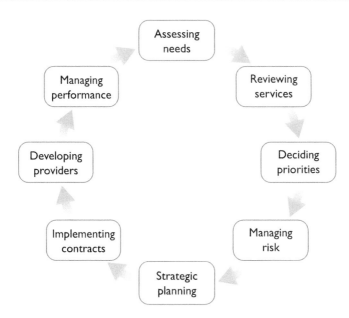

DESIGN OF CLINICAL COMMISSIONING GROUPS

- ▶ Membership bodies
- ▶ Clinically led
  - GP practices and other healthcare professionals
- ▶ Independent, and accountable to the Secretary of State for Health through NHS England
- ▶ Responsive to the health needs of their local populations
- ▶ Responsible for approximately two thirds of the NHS budget

GOVERNANCE OF CLINICAL COMMISSIONING GROUPS

- ▶ Governing body
  - Accountable Officer
  - Chief Finance Officer
  - Registered nurse
  - Secondary care specialist
  - Lay members
  - Often additional members
- ▶ Individual constitution

SERVICES OF CLINICAL COMMISSIONING GROUPS

- ▶ Locally commissioned services
  - Secondary care
  - Community services
  - Local public health services
  - Mental health
  - Rehabilitation services

SUPPORT FOR CLINICAL COMMISSIONING GROUPS

- ▶ Commissioning Support Units
  - Transactional commissioning
    - Market management
    - Contract negotiation
    - Healthcare procurement
    - Information analysis
    - Risk stratification

- Transformational commissioning
  - Service redesign
► Clinical Senates
  - Advisory groups of experts from across health and social care
    - Core Clinical Senate Council
    - Wider Clinical Senate Assembly
► Strategic Clinical Networks
  - Addressing priority service areas
    - Oncological
    - Cardiovascular
    - Maternity, children, young people
    - Mental health, dementia, neurological
  - Bringing together those who commission, provide and use services
  - Supporting effective service delivery

COMMISSIONING TRENDS

► Key changes
  - Joint working at a local level
  - Population and place based approaches
  - Integrated commissioning at a local level

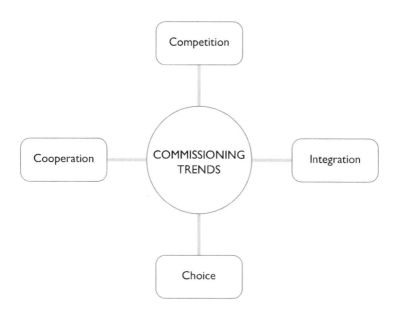

RIGHT OF CHOICE

- ▶ NHS main website
  - Health website with quality information and service directories
- ▶ NHS e-Referral Service
  - Location
  - Services
  - Consultants
  - Performance
  - Reputation
  - Visiting policies
  - Waiting times
  - Parking facilities
  - Patients' comments
  - Booking facility

- ▶ Complaints system in case of denied choice
  - Referring doctor
  - Local Healthwatch
  - CCG
  - NHS England
  - NHS Improvement
  - Ombudsman

PATIENT CHOICE AND COMPLAINTS SYSTEM

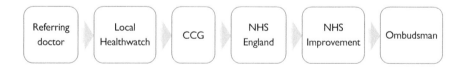

HEALTH AND WELLBEING BOARDS

- ▶ Members
  - Local authorities
  - Clinical commissioning groups

- Local Healthwatch
- Director of Children's Social Services
- Director of Adult Social Services
- Director of Public Health

► Functions

- Assessment of the local needs
- Promotion of integration, partnership and a joint health and wellbeing strategy across an area
- Involvement in the commissioning process

13 HEALTHCARE SERVICES

CHAPTER OVERVIEW

- ▶ **HEALTHCARE SERVICES**
- ▶ **NHS TRUSTS**
- ▶ **EMERGENCY CARE**
- ▶ **PUBLIC HEALTH**
- ▶ **PATIENT PROMISES**
- ▶ **SERVICE STANDARDS**
- ▶ **ORGANISATIONAL PROFESSIONALISM**

HEALTHCARE SERVICES

- ▶ Locally commissioned services
  - Secondary care
    - Hospital care, treatment centres
  - Community services
    - Allied health professionals, community nursing services, health visitors, community midwives
  - Local public health services
  - Mental health
  - Rehabilitation services
- ▶ Nationally commissioned services
  - Primary care
    - Medical, dental, pharmacy and optical services
  - Specialised healthcare
    - Low-volume, high-cost, centralised and specialised services
  - Immunisation, children, screening, prevention
  - Military healthcare
  - Offender healthcare

NHS TRUSTS

	NHS Foundation Trust	NHS Trust
Government involvement	Not directed by government	Directed by government
Financial regulation	NHS Improvement (formerly Monitor)	NHS Improvement (formerly Trust Development Authority)
Quality	Care Quality Commission	Care Quality Commission
Finance	Free to make financial decisions according to an agreed framework set out in law and by regulators Can retain operating surpluses Can vary staff pay from nationally agreed terms and conditions Can establish private companies	Financially accountable to government

EMERGENCY CARE

▶ GP out-of-hours services
▶ Urgent care: 111
▶ Emergency care: 999
▶ Accident and emergency departments
▶ Ambulance services
▶ Trauma services
▶ Critical care

PUBLIC HEALTH

▶ Domains
  ● Health protection
    ▪ E.g. disease outbreak prevention
  ● Health improvement
    ▪ E.g. health promotion, screening services
  ● Information
    ▪ E.g. research, development
  ● Operations
    ▪ E.g. national microbiology unit

▶ Goals
- Increased healthy life expectancy
- Reduced differences in life expectancy and healthy life expectancy between communities

PATIENT PROMISES

▶ Patients' needs always come first.

▶ A clean and safe hospital with comfortable and modern facilities
▶ A helpful, caring and respectful attitude
▶ An approachable and responsive team who listen to patients and involve patients in decisions about their care
▶ A flexible, reliable and punctual service
▶ A competent and skilled workforce to maintain and improve health

SERVICE STANDARDS

▶ Competence
▶ Communication
▶ Compassion
▶ Courtesy

ORGANISATIONAL PROFESSIONALISM

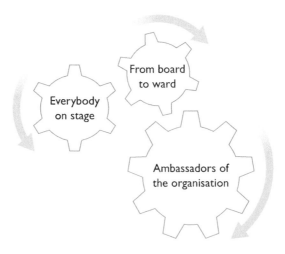

14 HEALTHCARE INFRASTRUCTURE

CHAPTER OVERVIEW

- ▶ **INFRASTRUCTURE LEGISLATION**
- ▶ **INFRASTRUCTURE MANAGEMENT**
- ▶ **INFRASTRUCTURE ASSESSMENT**
- ▶ **INFRASTRUCTURE SAFETY**
- ▶ **INFRASTRUCTURE RISKS**
- ▶ **INFRASTRUCTURE INCIDENTS**

INFRASTRUCTURE LEGISLATION

- ▶ Building Control Regulations
- ▶ Fire Safety Risk Assessment
- ▶ Regulatory Reform (Fire Safety) Order
- ▶ Control of Substances Hazardous to Health (COSHH) Regulations
- ▶ Management of Health and Safety at Work Regulations

INFRASTRUCTURE MANAGEMENT

- ▶ Responsible lead
- ▶ Maintenance team
- ▶ Local tradespeople

INFRASTRUCTURE ASSESSMENT

- ▶ Why should it be assessed?
- ▶ Who should assess it?
- ▶ Whose risk should be assessed?
- ▶ What should be assessed?
- ▶ When should it be assessed?

INFRASTRUCTURE SAFETY

▶ Hazardous substances
▶ Fire safety
▶ Infection control
▶ Security against intruders
▶ Protection from harm
▶ Security of property

INFRASTRUCTURE RISKS

▶ Identifying and controlling risks
▶ Setting up guidelines and reviewing them regularly
▶ Informing and training employees

INFRASTRUCTURE INCIDENTS

▶ Where
  • Health and Safety Executive
▶ What
  • Death cases
  • Major injuries
  • Accidents resulting in more than three days' absence
  • Certain diseases
  • Dangerous occurrences

15 HEALTHCARE REGULATION

CHAPTER OVERVIEW

- ► HEALTHCARE OFFICIALS
- ► CARE QUALITY COMMISSION
- ► NHS IMPROVEMENT
- ► MONITOR
- ► TRUST DEVELOPMENT AUTHORITY
- ► NHS CONFEDERATION
- ► NHS PROVIDERS
- ► OTHER REGULATORS
- ► PROFESSIONAL REGULATION
- ► GENERAL MEDICAL COUNCIL 'GOOD MEDICAL PRACTICE'
- ► DOMAIN 1: KNOWLEDGE, SKILLS AND PERFORMANCE
- ► DOMAIN 2: SAFETY AND QUALITY
- ► DOMAIN 3: COMMUNICATION, PARTNERSHIP AND TEAMWORK
- ► DOMAIN 4: MAINTAINING TRUST
- ► GENERAL MEDICAL COUNCIL 'GENERIC PROFESSIONAL CAPABILITIES FRAMEWORK'
- ► REVALIDATION
- ► ACCOUNTABILITY
- ► DECENTRALISATION
- ► BOARDS
- ► STANDARDS FOR MEMBERS OF BOARDS
- ► SEVEN PRINCIPLES OF PUBLIC LIFE
- ► BOARD COMMITTEES
- ► FOUNDATION TRUST BOARDS
- ► HEALTHWATCH
- ► ENGAGEMENT OF PATIENTS AND THE PUBLIC

HEALTHCARE OFFICIALS

- ▶ Secretary of State for Health
  - Overall responsibility for the work of the Department of Health
- ▶ Chief Medical Officer
  - Government's principal medical and scientific adviser
  - Professional lead for
    - ▪ Doctors in England
    - ▪ All Directors of Public Health in local government
- ▶ National Medical Director
  - Clinical policy, strategy, outcomes, leadership and innovation
- ▶ Chief Nursing Officer
  - Quality improvements in patient safety and patient experience
  - Professional lead for
    - ▪ Nurses
    - ▪ Midwives
- ▶ Chief Professional Officers
  - Chief Scientific Officer
  - Chief Dental Officer
  - Chief Pharmaceutical Officer
  - Chief Health Professions Officer
    - ▪ Expert advice across the health system

CARE QUALITY COMMISSION

- ▶ Independent regulator of health and social care
- ▶ Registration and inspection of all hospitals, care homes, GP surgeries and dental practices
  - Driving improvement
  - Putting patients first
  - Championing patients' rights
  - Remedying bad practice
  - Gathering expertise
- ▶ Enforcement powers if the fundamental standards of safety and quality are not met
  - Issuing warnings
  - Restricting service provision

- Issuing penalty notice
- Suspending service registration
- Prosecuting provider
▶ Primary values of the Care Quality Commission
  - Excellence
  - Caring
  - Integrity
  - Teamwork

NHS IMPROVEMENT

▶ Single oversight framework with aligned national bodies
  - Monitor
  - Trust Development Authority
  - Patient Safety
  - National Reporting and Learning System
  - Advancing Change Team
  - Intensive Support Teams
▶ Strong coherence with the provider accountability structure

MONITOR

▶ Now NHS Improvement
▶ Formerly
  - Financial regulator of foundation trusts
  - Made sure that foundation trusts were well led and well run
  - Made sure that the payment system promoted quality and efficiency

TRUST DEVELOPMENT AUTHORITY

▶ Now NHS Improvement
▶ Formerly
  - Financial regulator of trusts
  - Transition into foundation status
  - Monitoring performance
  - Assuring quality

NHS CONFEDERATION

▶ Authentic voice of NHS leadership

▶ Membership body that brings together and speaks on behalf of the whole health and care system

  • Helps the NHS to guarantee high standards for patients and best value for taxpayers

  • Influences health policy and represents members' views to government, parliament, policymakers and the public

  • Makes sense of the health system and healthcare providers with information and publications

  • Supports the whole health industry with the help of the NHS Employers organisation

NHS PROVIDERS

▶ Membership organisation and trade association for the NHS acute, ambulance, community and mental health services

OTHER REGULATORS

▶ General Medical Council

▶ General Dental Council

▶ General Pharmaceutical Council

▶ General Optical Council

▶ Nursing and Midwifery Council

▶ Health and Care Professions Council

PROFESSIONAL REGULATION

▶ Education

▶ Training

▶ Continuing professional development

▶ Registration

▶ Revalidation

▶ Setting standards
▶ Protecting patients
▶ Maintaining confidence in the system
▶ Determining the fitness to practise

Professional regulation			
Setting standards	Protecting patients	Maintaining confidence in the system	Determining the fitness to practise

GENERAL MEDICAL COUNCIL 'GOOD MEDICAL PRACTICE'

▶ Doctors are personally accountable for their professional practice and must always be prepared to justify their decisions and actions.

▶ An evidence base and a value base should substantiate all decisions and actions.

▶ Four domains of a doctor's duty
  • Domain 1: Knowledge, skills and performance
  • Domain 2: Safety and quality
  • Domain 3: Communication, partnership and teamwork
  • Domain 4: Maintaining trust

DOMAIN 1: KNOWLEDGE, SKILLS AND PERFORMANCE

▶ Make the care of your patient your first concern.
▶ Provide a good standard of practice and care.
  • Keep your professional knowledge and skills up to date.
  • Recognise and work within the limits of your competence.

DOMAIN 2: SAFETY AND QUALITY

▶ Take prompt action if you think that patient safety, dignity or comfort is being compromised.

▶ Protect and promote the health of patients and the public.

DOMAIN 3: COMMUNICATION, PARTNERSHIP AND TEAMWORK

▶ Treat patients as individuals and respect their dignity.
  • Treat patients politely and considerately.
  • Respect patients' right to confidentiality.
▶ Work in partnership with patients.
  • Listen to, and respond to, their concerns and preferences.
  • Give patients the information they want or need in a way they can understand.
  • Respect patients' right to reach decisions with you about their treatment and care.
  • Support patients in caring for themselves to improve and maintain their health.
▶ Work with colleagues in the ways that best serve patients' interests.

DOMAIN 4: MAINTAINING TRUST

▶ Be honest and open and act with integrity.
▶ Never discriminate unfairly against patients or colleagues.
▶ Never abuse your patients' trust in you or the public's trust in the profession.

GENERAL MEDICAL COUNCIL
'GENERIC PROFESSIONAL CAPABILITIES FRAMEWORK'

▶ Nine domains
  • Domain 1: Professional values and behaviours
  • Domain 2: Professional skills
  • Domain 3: Professional knowledge
  • Domain 4: Capabilities in health promotion and illness prevention
  • Domain 5: Capabilities in leadership and team working

- Domain 6: Capabilities in patient safety and quality improvement
- Domain 7: Capabilities in safeguarding vulnerable groups
- Domain 8: Capabilities in education and training
- Domain 9: Capabilities in research and scholarship

REVALIDATION

▶ Part of the system of measures to
- Promote safety and quality
- Ensure all medical practice is conducted in a governed system
  - Doctors 'up to date'
  - Doctors 'fit to practise'
  - Doctors 'safe'
  - Doctors 'competent'

▶ All doctors who have GMC registration with a licence to practise are legally required to revalidate.
- Every five years
- Annual appraisal process

▶ Important GMC guidance
- 'Continuing professional development – Guidance for all doctors'
- 'Effective governance to support medical revalidation – A handbook for boards and governing bodies'
- 'Generic professional capabilities framework'
- 'Good medical practice'
- 'Good medical practice framework for appraisal and revalidation'
- 'Guidance for doctors – Requirements for revalidation and maintaining your licence'
- 'Guidance on supporting information for appraisal and revalidation'
- 'The GMC protocol for making revalidation recommendations'

▶ Important Academy of Medical Royal Colleges guidance
- 'Supporting information for appraisal and revalidation'

▶ Important supporting information
- Continuing professional development
- Quality improvement activity

- Significant events
- Multi source feedback
- Compliments and complaints

▶ The Medical Director is usually the responsible officer of the designated body.

ACCOUNTABILITY

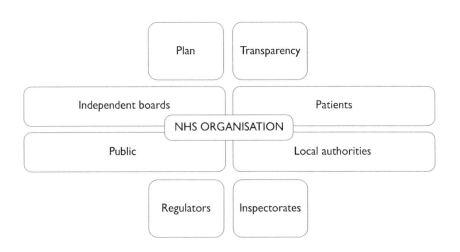

DECENTRALISATION

▶ Local leadership
▶ Local autonomy
▶ Local accountability

BOARDS

▶ Members
- Non-executives (subject matter experience)
  ▪ Chair (overall leadership)
- Executives (specific responsibility areas)
  ▪ Chief Executive (accountable officer)

▶ Role
  ● Formulating the strategy
  ● Controlling the organisation
  ● Shaping the culture
▶ Interactions
  ● Patients
  ● Public
  ● Staff
  ● Stakeholders
  ● Regulators

STANDARDS FOR MEMBERS OF BOARDS

▶ Personal behaviour
▶ Technical competence
▶ Business practices

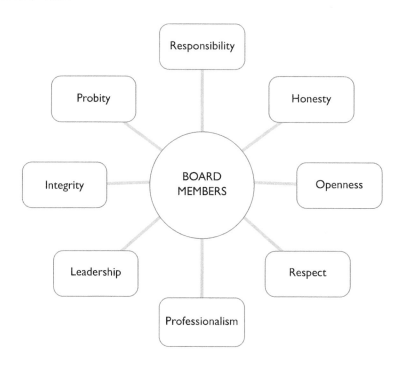

SEVEN PRINCIPLES OF PUBLIC LIFE

▶ Nolan principles for holders of public office
- Selflessness
- Integrity
- Objectivity
- Accountability
- Openness
- Honesty
- Leadership

BOARD COMMITTEES

▶ Audit committee
▶ Remuneration committee
▶ Clinical governance committee
▶ Risk management committee

FOUNDATION TRUST BOARDS

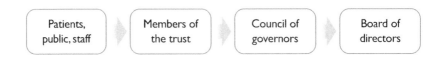

▶ Board of directors
- Trust management including day-to-day operation and business plan
  - Non-executive directors appointed by the governors
  - Executive directors appointed by the non-executive directors

HEALTHWATCH

▶ Independent consumer champion organisation
▶ Represents the public's view on healthcare

- ▶ Local and national levels
  - • Local Healthwatch
    - ▪ Supports patients
    - ▪ Feeds intelligence to Healthwatch England
    - ▪ Influences commissioning
  - • Healthwatch England
    - ▪ Provides leadership to Local Healthwatch
    - ▪ Provides advice to the Secretary of State for Health, NHS England, NHS Improvement and the local authorities
    - ▪ Proposes investigations of poor services

ENGAGEMENT OF PATIENTS AND THE PUBLIC

- ▶ 'Patients first and foremost'
- ▶ 'Patients at the heart of everything'
- ▶ 'No decision about me, without me'
- ▶ 'The NHS belongs to the people'

- ▶ Involvement in planning, delivering and evaluating services
- ▶ Involvement in constructive dialogues, relationships and partnerships

- ▶ Healthwatch
  - • Independent national consumer champion organisation
  - • Represents the public's view on healthcare
  - • Works to get services right
- ▶ Patient Advice and Liaison Service
  - • Advises about local health services and local support groups
  - • Helps with complaints procedures
  - • Highlights gaps in services and makes recommendations for action

- ▶ Patient representation groups
- ▶ Comments, compliments, complaints and concerns
- ▶ Public pressure groups

16 HEALTHCARE INSPECTION

CHAPTER OVERVIEW

▶ **CQC HEALTHCARE ROLE**
▶ **CQC HEALTHCARE STRATEGY**
▶ **CQC INSPECTION STANDARDS**
▶ **CQC INSPECTION TYPES**
▶ **CQC INSPECTION APPROACH**
▶ **CQC INSPECTION RATING**
▶ **CQC ENFORCEMENT POWERS**
▶ **CQC QUALITY IMPACT**
▶ **NHS IMPROVEMENT STRATEGY**
▶ **SINGLE OVERSIGHT FRAMEWORK**
▶ **WELL LED FRAMEWORK**

CQC HEALTHCARE ROLE

▶ Independent regulator of health and social care

▶ Registration and inspection of all hospitals, care homes, GP surgeries and dental practices

▶ Registering
▶ Monitoring
▶ Inspecting
▶ Rating
▶ Reporting
▶ Acting

▶ Improving

▶ Gathering information from many sources
- Providers
- Staff
- Patients
- Authorities
- Healthwatch
- Ombudsmen
- Complaints
- Whistleblowing
- Concerns
- Inspection
- Documents
- Records

CQC HEALTHCARE STRATEGY

▶ Ambition
- A more targeted, responsive and collaborative approach
▶ Priorities
- Encouraging improvement, innovation and sustainability
- Delivering an intelligence driven approach to regulation
- Promoting a single shared view of quality
- Improving efficiency, effectiveness and expertise

CQC INSPECTION STANDARDS

▶ Standards of safety and quality
- Skills, qualifications and experience of staff
- Size, layout and design of place
- Policies, systems and procedures of provider
▶ NICE Social Care Quality Standards

CQC INSPECTION TYPES

▶ Comprehensive inspections
▶ Focused inspections

CQC INSPECTION APPROACH

▶ Key questions
- Is the service safe?
- Is the service effective?
- Is the service caring?
- Is the service responsive?
- Is the service well-led?

▶ Is the service safe?
- Focus: Safeguarding issues

▶ Is the service effective?
- Focus: Health outcome

▶ Is the service caring?
- Focus: Service culture

▶ Is the service responsive?
- Focus: Timely reaction

▶ Is the service well-led?
- Focus: Organisational structure

▶ Key lines of enquiry
- Five key questions broken down into further detailed questions
  - Consistent approach for all inspections

▶ Is it a personalised, high quality, safe service?
  • Objective measures
  • Evidence
  • Professional judgement

▶ Core services
  • Urgent and emergency services
  • Medical care including older people's care
  • Surgery
  • Gynaecology
  • Intensive and critical care
  • End of life care
  • Services for children and young people
  • Outpatient services and imaging

CQC INSPECTION RATING

▶ Rating for each of the key questions and for each of the core services plus an overall rating for the whole service
  • Outstanding
  • Good
  • Requires improvement
  • Inadequate

CQC ENFORCEMENT POWERS

▶ Issuing warnings
▶ Restricting service provision
▶ Issuing penalty notice
▶ Suspending service registration
▶ Prosecuting provider

CQC QUALITY IMPACT

▶ The CQC puts safety and quality at the heart of the ratings system.

▶ The CQC has developed a framework for safety and quality which is unique anywhere in the world.

▶ The CQC deserves great credit for overhauling healthcare regulation and defining healthcare standards.

NHS IMPROVEMENT STRATEGY

▶ Single Oversight Framework
  - Supporting providers to improve to attain and/or maintain a CQC 'good' or 'outstanding' rating
▶ Well Led Framework

SINGLE OVERSIGHT FRAMEWORK

▶ Five key themes
  - Quality of care
  - Finance and use of resources
  - Operational performance
  - Strategic change
  - Leadership and improvement capability
▶ Provider support need
  - No: Maximum autonomy
  - Yes, with some support needs: Providers offered targeted support
  - Yes, with significant concerns: Providers receiving mandated support
  - Yes, with major/complex concerns: Special measures

WELL LED FRAMEWORK

▶ Key lines of enquiry
  - Leadership capacity? Leadership capability?
  - Clear vision? Credible strategy?
  - Culture?
  - Responsibilities? Roles? Accountability?
  - Risks? Issues? Performance?
  - Information?
  - Staff engaged? Patients involved?
  - Learning systems? Improvement processes?

17 HEALTHCARE REVIEWS

CHAPTER OVERVIEW

- ► PATIENT SAFETY PROBLEMS
- ► MAJOR REVIEWS OF PATIENT SAFETY
- ► THE DARZI REPORT
- ► THE FRANCIS REPORT
- ► THE KEOGH REPORT
- ► THE BERWICK REPORT
- ► THE GREENAWAY REPORT

PATIENT SAFETY PROBLEMS

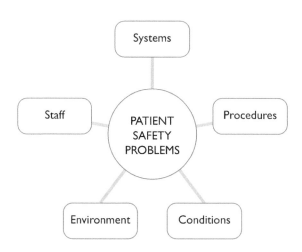

MAJOR REVIEWS OF PATIENT SAFETY

- ► The Darzi Report (June 2008)
- ► The Francis Report (February 2013)

▶ The Keogh Report (July 2013)
▶ The Berwick Report (August 2013)
▶ The Greenaway Report (October 2013)

THE DARZI REPORT

▶ 'High quality care for all'
▶ Focuses on improving the quality of care in the NHS
  • Health promotion
  • Personalised care
  • Quality monitoring
  • Better training
  • More integration
  • NHS Constitution

THE FRANCIS REPORT

▶ 'Mid Staffordshire Public Inquiry'
▶ Focuses on a broad range of issues relating to patient care and safety
  • Culture
  • Standards
  • Candour
  • Patients first
  • Compassionate care
  • Transparent information

THE KEOGH REPORT

▶ 'Quality of care and treatment'
▶ Focuses on different factors leading to high mortality
  • Patient experience
  • Safety
  • Workforce
  • Effectiveness
  • Leadership
  • Corporate governance

THE BERWICK REPORT

▶ 'A promise to learn – A commitment to act: Improving the safety of patients'
▶ Focuses on a system devoted to continual learning and improvement of patient care, top to bottom and end to end
  - Leadership
  - Staff
  - Patient and public involvement
  - Training and capacity building
  - Measurement and transparency
  - Structures and regulation

THE GREENAWAY REPORT

▶ 'Securing the future of excellent patient care'
▶ Focuses on a training structure for the future
  - Involving patients in training doctors
  - Balance between generalists and specialists
  - Broader approach to postgraduate training
  - Tension between service and training
  - More flexibility in medical training

18 HEALTHCARE GOVERNANCE

CHAPTER OVERVIEW

- ► **THEMES OF GOVERNANCE**
- ► **TYPES OF GOVERNANCE**
- ► **FORMAL DEFINITION OF CLINICAL GOVERNANCE**
- ► **KEY ATTRIBUTES OF CLINICAL GOVERNANCE**
- ► **MAIN COMPONENTS OF CLINICAL GOVERNANCE**

THEMES OF GOVERNANCE

- ► Purpose, roles, behaviours
- ► Principles
- ► Leadership, direction
- ► Relationships
- ► Transparency, reporting
- ► Outcomes
- ► Risk, compliance
- ► Effectiveness
- ► Safety, quality, innovation

TYPES OF GOVERNANCE

- ► Clinical governance
- ► Research governance
- ► Information governance
- ► Corporate governance

FORMAL DEFINITION OF CLINICAL GOVERNANCE

▶ Framework of systems, processes and controls which helps healthcare organisations demonstrate accountability for improving the quality of their services and safeguarding the standards of care

KEY ATTRIBUTES OF CLINICAL GOVERNANCE

▶ High standards
▶ Transparent responsibility and accountability
▶ Continuous improvement

```
┌─────────────────────────────────────────────────────────────┐
│                    Clinical governance                       │
└─────────────────────────────────────────────────────────────┘
┌──────────────────┐ ┌──────────────────────┐ ┌──────────────────────┐
│                  │ │ Transparent responsibility │ │                      │
│  High standards  │ │   and accountability   │ │ Continuous improvement │
└──────────────────┘ └──────────────────────┘ └──────────────────────┘
```

MAIN COMPONENTS OF CLINICAL GOVERNANCE

▶ Risk management
▶ Clinical audit
▶ Education and training
▶ Research and development
▶ Transparency
▶ Accountability
▶ Standards and compliance
▶ Compliments and complaints
▶ Clinical effectiveness
▶ Information management

19 HEALTHCARE RISKS

CHAPTER OVERVIEW

▶ **HEALTHCARE RISKS**
▶ **RISK REGISTER**
▶ **RISK ANALYSIS**
▶ **RISK MANAGEMENT**

HEALTHCARE RISKS

▶ Healthcare risks
  - Risk is inevitable.
  - Risk can be quantified.
  - Risk can be managed.
  - Risk is reducible.

RISK REGISTER

▶ Risk register
  - Safety net for all staff
  - Identification and scoring of risks through a top-down and bottom-up process
  - Important basis for management decisions

RISK ANALYSIS

▶ Root cause analysis in case of a serious untoward incident
  - Five whys
  - Fishbone diagrams

- 4 Ms: Machines, manpower, materials, methods
- 4 Ps: People, place, policies, procedures
- 4 Ss: Skills, suppliers, surroundings, systems

RISK MANAGEMENT

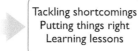

| Adverse incidents
Near misses
Malpractice
Wrongdoing | Tackling shortcomings
Putting things right
Learning lessons | Higher standards
Better quality |

| Auditing
Benchmarking
Feedback
Outcomes | Monitoring quality
Reviewing quality
Improving quality
Assuring quality |

20 HEALTHCARE SAFETY

CHAPTER OVERVIEW

▶ **PATIENT SAFETY**
▶ **SAFETY MONITORING**
▶ **SAFETY CULTURE**
▶ **HEALTHCARE SAFETY INVESTIGATION BRANCH (HSIB)**

PATIENT SAFETY

▶ Medicine
  • The right treatment to the right patient, via the right route, with the right dose, at the right time, with the right documentation
▶ Surgery
  • The correct surgery on the correct patient, with the correct items, on the correct body part, at the correct procedure site, after a correct time out

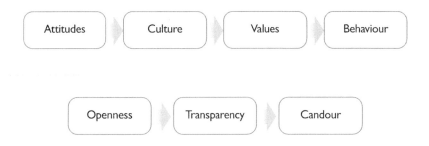

| Attitudes | Culture | Values | Behaviour |

| Openness | Transparency | Candour |

SAFETY MONITORING

| Safety thermometer | Healthcare associated infections | Never events | Central alerting system |

SAFETY CULTURE

▶ Learning from failings
- Analysing the organisation's safety regulations
- Developing a sustainable action plan
- Intensifying the patient safety initiatives

▶ Learning from failings
- Aligning the organisation around safety
  - Developing a high reliability organisation
- Aligning the organisation around transparency

▶ Ownership of safety lies with senior leaders and frontline staff alike.
- Connecting board and ward
  - Encouraging vigilance
  - Empowering staff
  - Involving patients
  - Resolving concerns
  - Providing feedback
▶ Safety should have the very highest priority across the entire organisation.

▶ People's intrinsic desire to do their best is the cornerstone of a robust safety culture.
- It is not about a compliance mindset.
- It is not about passing CQC tests.
▶ Everyone must uphold safety oriented behaviours and processes and encourage others to do the same.

HEALTHCARE SAFETY INVESTIGATION BRANCH (HSIB)

▶ Expert advisory group
- Funded by DoH
- Hosted by NHSI
- Independent from CQC

▶ Improving safety through effective and independent investigations which do not apportion blame or liability

- Focusing on learning
- Identifying common themes and patterns
- Developing meaningful and influential recommendations
- Developing skills and raising standards
- Driving positive change

▶ Main operating principles

- Independence in judgement
- Expertise
- Objectivity
- Transparency
- Learning for improvement

21 HEALTHCARE QUALITY

CHAPTER OVERVIEW

▶ QUALITY DEFINITION
▶ PATIENT SAFETY
▶ CLINICAL EFFECTIVENESS
▶ PATIENT EXPERIENCE
▶ QUALITY MODEL
▶ QUALITY ELEMENTS
▶ QUALITY FOCUS
▶ QUALITY DIMENSIONS
▶ QUALITY INDICATORS
▶ QUALITY CATALYSTS
▶ QUALITY MEASUREMENT
▶ QUALITY ASSURANCE
▶ QUALITY IMPROVEMENT
▶ QUALITY GOVERNANCE
▶ QUALITY CULTURE
▶ QUALITY ACCOUNT
▶ NATIONAL QUALITY BOARD (NQB)
▶ NATIONAL INSTITUTE FOR HEALTH AND CARE EXCELLENCE (NICE)
▶ NATIONAL SERVICE FRAMEWORKS (NSFS)
▶ NHS OUTCOMES FRAMEWORK (NHS OF)
▶ CARE QUALITY COMMISSION (CQC)
▶ CHIEF INSPECTOR OF HOSPITALS
▶ QUALITY SURVEILLANCE GROUPS (QSGS)
▶ COMMISSIONING FOR QUALITY AND INNOVATION (CQUIN)
▶ QUALITY, INNOVATION, PRODUCTIVITY AND PREVENTION (QIPP)

▶ **QUALITY PREMIUM (QP)**
▶ **QUALITY AND OUTCOMES FRAMEWORK (QOF)**
▶ **PATIENT SURVEYS**
▶ **PATIENT REPORTED OUTCOME MEASURES (PROMS)**
▶ **FRIENDS AND FAMILY TEST (FFT)**

QUALITY DEFINITION

▶ Excellence in patient safety, clinical effectiveness and patient experience

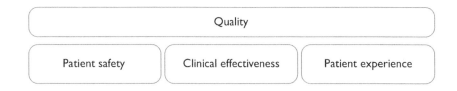

PATIENT SAFETY

▶ 'Good services help to keep me safe.'

CLINICAL EFFECTIVENESS

▶ 'Good services make me feel better and more independent.'

PATIENT EXPERIENCE

▶ 'Good services treat me well.'

QUALITY MODEL

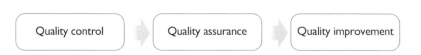

QUALITY ELEMENTS

▶ A caring culture, a professional commitment and a strong leadership

QUALITY FOCUS

▶ Narrowing the gap between the best and the worst, while raising the bar higher for everyone

QUALITY DIMENSIONS

▶ Safe
▶ Effective
▶ Efficient
▶ Consistent
▶ Evidence based
▶ Patient centred
▶ Prompt
▶ Timely
▶ Integrated
▶ Equitable

QUALITY INDICATORS

▶ Numerous indicators generally accepted as effective measures of care quality
  • Selected with the Royal Colleges
  • Aligned to the five domains in the NHS Outcomes Framework
  • Applied in a local setting

▶ Mortality ratio
▶ Infection rate
▶ Adverse incidents
▶ Timeliness of service delivery
▶ Length of hospital stay
▶ Patient feedback
▶ Staff contentedness
▶ Financial performance

QUALITY CATALYSTS

▶ Leadership
▶ Governance
▶ Creativity
▶ Learning
▶ Communication skills
▶ Staff empowerment
▶ Outside perspective
▶ Improvement plan
▶ Safety culture
▶ Change management
▶ Cultural change
▶ Systems thinking
▶ Patient involvement
▶ Public engagement
▶ CQC inspections
▶ Values
▶ Vision
▶ Resilience
▶ Tenacity

QUALITY MEASUREMENT

▶ Approach 1: Equality, human rights, diversity
▶ Approach 2: Is it safe? Is it effective? Is it caring? Is it responsive? Is it well-led?
▶ Approach 3: Safety, patient experience, effectiveness

▶ Approach 4: Outcome-based frameworks
▶ Approach 5: Standards-based frameworks

▶ Approach 6: Feedback
▶ Approach 7: Benchmarks

QUALITY ASSURANCE

▶ Approach: Monitoring system

QUALITY IMPROVEMENT

▶ Approach 1: Plan – do – check – act
▶ Approach 2: Where are we now? – Where do we want to be? – How will we get there? – When will we get there?

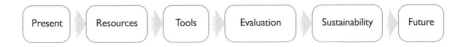

QUALITY GOVERNANCE

▶ Combination of structures and processes at and below board level to lead on organisation-wide quality performance
  • Achieving required standards
  • Delivering best practice
  • Planning continuous improvement
  • Investigating substandard performance
  • Managing quality risks

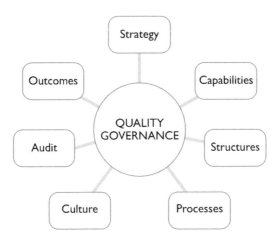

QUALITY CULTURE

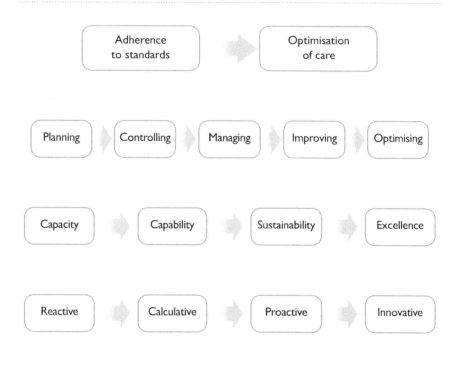

QUALITY ACCOUNT

▶ Annual quality account
- Statement of accountability
- Quality of services
- Results from inspections
- Priorities for improvement

NATIONAL QUALITY BOARD (NQB)

▶ Strategic oversight and leadership in quality across the NHS
▶ Coordinated leadership for quality on behalf of the national bodies
- Department of Health
- Public Health England
- NHS England
- Care Quality Commission

- NHS Improvement
- National Institute for Health and Care Excellence
▶ Alignment of the systems for quality throughout the NHS

NATIONAL INSTITUTE FOR HEALTH AND CARE EXCELLENCE (NICE)

▶ National guidance and advice to improve health and social care
- Produces evidence based guidance
- Sets legally binding quality standards
- Provides several informational services

NATIONAL SERVICE FRAMEWORKS (NSFS)

▶ Policy set by the NHS
▶ Long term strategies and evidence based programmes setting quality standards and specifying services that should be available for a particular condition or care group across the whole NHS
▶ Offers strategies and targeted support

NHS OUTCOMES FRAMEWORK (NHS OF)

▶ Overview of NHS national performance
▶ Mechanism to hold NHS England to account
▶ Catalyst for NHS quality improvement

Effectiveness	Domain 1	Preventing people from dying prematurely
	Domain 2	Enhancing quality of life for people with long term conditions
	Domain 3	Helping people to recover from episodes of ill health or following injury
Experience	Domain 4	Ensuring that people have a positive experience of care
Safety	Domain 5	Treating and caring for people in a safe environment and protecting them from avoidable harm

CARE QUALITY COMMISSION (CQC)

- ▶ Independent regulator of health and social care
- ▶ Registration and inspection of all hospitals, care homes, GP surgeries and dental practices
  - Driving improvement
  - Putting patients first
  - Championing patients' rights
  - Remedying bad practice
  - Gathering expertise
- ▶ Enforcement powers if the fundamental standards of safety and quality are not met
  - Issuing warnings
  - Restricting service provision
  - Issuing penalty notice
  - Suspending service registration
  - Prosecuting provider
- ▶ Primary values of the Care Quality Commission
  - Excellence
  - Caring
  - Integrity
  - Teamwork

CHIEF INSPECTOR OF HOSPITALS

- ▶ Assesses the performance of NHS hospitals
  - Inspects the hospitals concerned without announcement
  - Identifies poor care without any hesitation
- ▶ Is the whistleblower of the nation

QUALITY SURVEILLANCE GROUPS (QSGS)

- ▶ Forums of commissioners, regulators and others who share information on quality to spot signs of problems and take action to prevent more serious quality failures
  - Local QSGs
  - Regional QSGs

COMMISSIONING FOR QUALITY AND INNOVATION (CQUIN)

▶ Framework supporting improvements in the quality of services and the patterns of care
  - Delivering clinical quality improvements and driving transformational change
  - All schemes to include national goals
    - Using the friends and family test
    - Applying the safety thermometer
    - Improving dementia care quality
    - Reducing the complications from venous thromboembolism
  - Part of income conditional on quality and innovation

QUALITY, INNOVATION, PRODUCTIVITY AND PREVENTION (QIPP)

▶ Programme designed to identify savings which can be reinvested in the health service and improve the care quality

QUALITY PREMIUM (QP)

▶ Quality premium payment for clinical commissioning groups if they achieve the required improvements in service quality

QUALITY AND OUTCOMES FRAMEWORK (QOF)

▶ Voluntary incentive scheme to encourage high quality services in general practice
▶ Four domains of the national standards
  - Clinical standards for chronic disease
  - Public health and primary prevention
  - Quality and productivity
  - Experience of patients

PATIENT SURVEYS

▶ Patients have a voice and patients have a choice.
  - Increased awareness

- Higher expectations (mentality of entitlement?)
- Reduced tolerance

▶ Contents
- What people need and expect from the NHS
- How well the NHS has responded to their needs and expectations

▶ Aims
- Monitor patients' experience nationally
- Assess users' experience for performing inspections, reviews and ratings
- Improve local care quality

▶ Programmes
- National patient survey programme
- General Practitioner patient survey
- NHS website
- Local surveys

▶ Others
- Patient stories
- Patient complaints
- Suggestion cards
- Mystery shoppers

PATIENT REPORTED OUTCOME MEASURES (PROMS)

▶ Method of collecting information on the quality of care from the patient's perspective
▶ Examples
- Hip replacement
- Knee replacement
- Groin hernia surgery
- Varicose vein surgery

FRIENDS AND FAMILY TEST (FFT)

▶ 'How likely are you to recommend our ward/A&E department to friends and family if they needed similar care or treatment?'

22 HEALTHCARE AUDIT

CHAPTER OVERVIEW

AUDIT DEFINITION

► Tool for quality
► Quality improvement through a systematic review (prospective, retrospective) of local performance against national criteria (standards, benchmarks) plus a change process
► Method of improvement

- Clinical research
  - Creates new knowledge
- Clinical audit
  - Analyses collected data against agreed standards of best practice
- Service evaluation
  - Assesses service effectiveness

AUDIT AIMS

- Driving quality improvement
- Driving quality standards
- Decreasing incidents
- Decreasing variation

AUDIT ROLE

- Role of audit in healthcare
  - Quality assurance
  - Clinical governance
  - Clinical effectiveness
  - Cost effectiveness
  - Evidence based medicine
  - Research
  - Training
  - Appraisal
  - Revalidation

AUDIT ADVANTAGES

- Improved care quality
- Improved team working
- Improved working environment
- Openness to change
- Basis for guidelines
- Reassurance for patients
- Fewer medical complications
- Fewer patient complaints
- Fewer patient claims

AUDIT BENEFICIARIES

▶ Patients
▶ Public
▶ Healthcare professionals
▶ Healthcare management

AUDIT TRIGGERS

▶ Recurrent problems
▶ Direct observation
▶ Adverse incidents
▶ Near misses
▶ Patient experience
▶ Patient feedback
▶ National regulations
▶ National guidelines
▶ Local regulations
▶ Local guidelines

AUDIT TOPICS

▶ Official selection criteria
  • Department of Health
  • National Institute for Health and Care Excellence
  • Medical Royal Colleges
▶ Traditional selection criteria
  • High volume
  • High risk
  • High impact
  • High cost
▶ Other selection criteria
  • Relevance of problem
  • Availability of standards, recommendations, targets or benchmarks
  • Amenability to change

AUDIT SKILLS

▶ Organisational skills
▶ Team working
▶ Project design
▶ Information technology
▶ Statistical methods
▶ Managerial skills

AUDIT MANAGEMENT

▶ Funding
▶ Support
  • Internal sources
    ▪ Clinical Audit Team
    ▪ Clinical Audit Department
  • External sources
    ▪ Royal Colleges
    ▪ National audit bodies
    ▪ King's Fund
▶ Timeline

AUDIT CYCLE

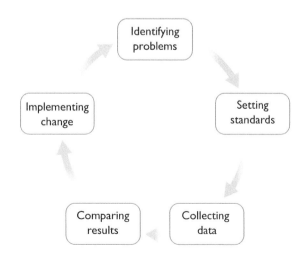

GENERAL RULES

▶ Audit should be a part of the broader quality improvement programme.

▶ Audit your own practice, not the practice of others.

▶ Audit should cross care boundaries and encompass the whole patient pathway.

IDENTIFYING PROBLEMS

▶ Selection of a topic
  • Impact?
  • Risk?
  • Volume?
  • Cost?
▶ Review of the literature
  • Previous audits?
  • Previous research?
  • Available guidelines?
  • Available standards?

SETTING STANDARDS

▶ Standard: Topic to be measured
  • Specific
  • Measurable
  • Achievable
  • Relevant
  • Timed
▶ Criterion: Measurement or yardstick
  • Clinical
  • Organisational
▶ Target: Percentage to be achieved

COLLECTING DATA

▶ Definition of population

▶ Definition of exceptions

▶ Definition of study period

▶ Definition of statistical methods

- Please note
  - Patient consent?
  - Ethics approval?
  - Data protection?
  - Patient confidentiality?

COMPARING RESULTS

▶ Comparison: Own data versus identified standards

- Standards met?
- Standards not met?
  - Analysis of reasons
  - Suggestions for improvement

▶ Outcome: Making sense of obtained results

- Care quality benefits?
- Patient satisfaction benefits?
- Cost effectiveness benefits?

▶ Presentation: Results from a clinical perspective

- Tables
- Charts
  - Pie charts
  - Bar charts
- Histograms
- Dashboards
  - Green: No action required
  - Amber: Action required
  - Red: Urgent action required

IMPLEMENTING CHANGE

▶ Action plan
- Implementing change
  - Responsible individuals
  - Appropriate teams
  - Monitoring method
  - Commencing date
  - Time frame
- Improving quality

▶ Re-audit schedule
- Further monitoring
  - Completing the first audit loop
  - Beginning the next audit loop
- Improving quality

CLINICAL AUDIT

▶ Important instrument of quality governance
- Improvement of services
- Information for patients
- Revalidation of clinicians

23 HEALTHCARE INCIDENTS

CHAPTER OVERVIEW

▶ **SAFETY INCIDENTS**
▶ **INCIDENT ANALYSIS**
▶ **INCIDENT MANAGEMENT**
▶ **INCIDENT PREVENTION**
▶ **NEVER EVENTS**

SAFETY INCIDENTS

▶ Events in which something has gone wrong, causing potential or actual harm

INCIDENT ANALYSIS

▶ Serious Incident Framework
▶ Structured methodology and analysis
▶ Root cause analysis
  • Key issues
  • Contributory factors
  • Underlying system issues
  • Key causal factors

▶ Away from acts and omissions of staff
▶ Towards origins and causes of incident

▶ Identifying underlying human factors to analyse the incident
  • Consistent, constructive and fair evaluation of the actions of staff involved in the incident

- Deliberate harm test
- Health test
- Foresight test
- Substitution test
- Mitigating circumstances test

▶ Using human factors principles to prevent future incidents

INCIDENT MANAGEMENT

▶ Reporting
▶ Investigating
▶ Involving patients and families
▶ Identifying causes of incident
▶ Learning
▶ Improving

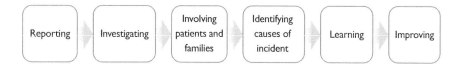

▶ Prompt reaction
▶ Professional reaction
▶ Precise reaction
▶ Positive reaction
▶ Proactive reaction

▶ Duty of candour
▶ Openness and transparency
▶ Learning, not blaming

INCIDENT PREVENTION

▶ Standardisation
▶ Training

▶ Minimising dependency on memory and attention
▶ Reducing reliance on protocols and policies

▶ Simplification
▶ Discipline
▶ Creating a safe and organised workplace
▶ Eliminating all redundant and unnecessary items

▶ Reducing waste in the thoughtflow
▶ Reducing waste in the workflow

▶ The cost of prevention is much less than the cost of harm.

NEVER EVENTS

▶ Serious, largely preventable and alarming adverse events in medicine
  • NHS Never Events List

▶ Main causes of never events
  • Lack of training
  • Incompetence
  • Overconfidence
  • Hubris
  • Laziness
  • Carelessness
  • Irresponsibility
  • Lack of standards

▶ Four actions to be taken following a never event
  • Apologising to patient
  • Reporting the event
  • Performing a root cause analysis
  • Waiving the directly related costs

24 HEALTHCARE SAFEGUARDING

CHAPTER OVERVIEW

- ▶ UNDERSTANDING SAFEGUARDING PRINCIPLES
- ▶ RECOGNISING SAFEGUARDING ISSUES
- ▶ IDENTIFYING ABUSE VICTIMS
- ▶ REALISING RISK FACTORS
- ▶ REPORTING SAFEGUARDING ISSUES
- ▶ WHISTLEBLOWING SAFEGUARDING ISSUES
- ▶ MANAGING SAFEGUARDING ISSUES
- ▶ EMBEDDING SAFEGUARDING AWARENESS
- ▶ APPLYING SAFEGUARDING PRINCIPLES

UNDERSTANDING SAFEGUARDING PRINCIPLES

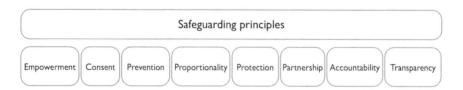

Safeguarding principles							
Empowerment	Consent	Prevention	Proportionality	Protection	Partnership	Accountability	Transparency

- ▶ A way of thinking
- ▶ A way of working

RECOGNISING SAFEGUARDING ISSUES

- ▶ Bad care
- ▶ Undermined dignity
- ▶ Maltreatment

- Harm
- Punitive responses to challenging behaviours
- Abuse
- Neglect
- Rigid routines
- Unhygienic environments

- Unchallenged superhero status
- Lone wolf mentality
- Unusual behaviour
- Arbitrary decisions

IDENTIFYING ABUSE VICTIMS

- Physical
- Psychological
- Sexual
- Neglect
- Discrimination
- Institutional
- Financial
- Legal

REALISING RISK FACTORS

- Low staffing levels
- High job stress
- Poor staff morale
- Insufficient policy awareness
- Inadequate leadership
- Weak management
- System problems
- Process failures
- Frail service users
- Mental health issues
- Geographically isolated services
- Neglected physical environment

REPORTING SAFEGUARDING ISSUES

▶ Safeguarding lead
▶ Safeguarding team
▶ Police
▶ Local commissioners
▶ Contract partners

WHISTLEBLOWING SAFEGUARDING ISSUES

▶ The Public Interest Disclosure Act protects whistleblowers who make disclosures about
  ● Criminal offence
  ● Breach of law
  ● Danger to the health and safety of any individual
  ● Miscarriage of justice
  ● Damaged environment
  ● Cover-up of information on any of the above matters

MANAGING SAFEGUARDING ISSUES

▶ Making records of all aspects of the issue
▶ Making notes at the time of the incident
▶ Recording facts and not opinions or even rumours
▶ Recording briefings and all meetings about safeguarding issues

▶ Before safeguarding and/or police investigation
  ● Allegations: Employer to follow disciplinary procedures (e.g. transfer, suspension of the person), to make accurate records, to cooperate with the responsible authorities and to review the service standards
▶ After safeguarding and/or police investigation
  ● Allegations upheld, but not charged with a criminal offence: Employer to follow disciplinary procedures (e.g. warning, dismissal of the person) and to notify the Disclosure and Barring Service and the local safeguarding team
  ● Person arrested and charged with a criminal offence: Police to notify the Disclosure and Barring Service and the local safeguarding team

EMBEDDING SAFEGUARDING AWARENESS

▶ Informed staff
▶ Empowered patients
▶ Attentive relatives
▶ Constant awareness
▶ Continual vigilance

APPLYING SAFEGUARDING PRINCIPLES

▶ Empowerment
▶ Consent
▶ Prevention
▶ Proportionality
▶ Protection
▶ Partnership
▶ Accountability
▶ Transparency

▶ Away from process-led care towards patient-centred care
  • Personalisation agenda with patients having choice, flexibility and control over their care
    ▪ Safeguarding to be done with, not to, patients

25 HEALTHCARE COMPLAINTS

CHAPTER OVERVIEW

▶ PATIENT COMPLAINTS
▶ COMPLAINTS PROCEDURE
▶ COMPLAINTS INVESTIGATION
▶ COMPLAINTS IMPACT
▶ SAYING SORRY

PATIENT COMPLAINTS

▶ Four most common complaints
  - Poor communication
  - Poor attention to toileting needs
  - Poor attention to nutritional needs
  - Pain relief

COMPLAINTS PROCEDURE

▶ Local level: NHS
  - Quick, thorough and objective procedure
    ▪ Responsive to the complainant
    ▪ Fair to the health professional complained against
▶ Local level: Local Government Ombudsman
▶ National level: Parliamentary and Health Service Ombudsman

▶ Main principles of the complaints procedure
  - Listening
  - Responding
  - Improving

▶ Important aspects of the complaints procedure
  • Patients have 12 months from the event occurrence to complain.
  • Formal complaints must be acknowledged within 3 days.
  • Formal complaints must be kept for 10 years.
  • Complaint letters from patients must not be kept in their medical records.

COMPLAINTS INVESTIGATION

▶ Investigation of a complaint
  • Seriousness of issue
  • Likelihood of recurrence
  • Category of risk
  • Course of action

▶ Principles of the investigation
  • Open
  • Transparent
  • Logical
  • Rational
  • Accountable
  • Evidence based
  • Comprehensive
  • Proportionate
  • Timely
  • Expeditious
  • Fair

▶ Results of a complaint
  • Apology
  • Explanation
  • Improvement
  • Conciliation
  • Mediation
  • Arbitration
  • Reimbursement
  • Claim
  • Compensation

COMPLAINTS IMPACT

▶ Impact of complaints on staff
  • Positive
    ▪ Quality improvement
  • Negative
    ▪ Culture of fear
    ▪ Defensive medical practice
    ▪ Increase in costs
    ▪ Low workplace morale
    ▪ Leaving the profession
    ▪ Mental health problems

▶ In view of the impact of complaints procedures on staff, there must be
  • Safe space protection for staff during investigations into mistakes in care
  • Rapid resolutions of vexatious complaints and clear consequences for vexatious complainants

SAYING SORRY

▶ Meaningful apology for suffering and distress
▶ Sincere expression of sorrow and regret
  • Verbal and written
  • As soon as possible
  • Based solely upon facts
  • Open and truthful

▶ Key principles of saying sorry
  • Timeliness of apology
  • Disclosure
  • Information
  • Explanation
  • Support
  • Confidentiality
  • Continuity of care

▶ Saying sorry is not an admission of legal liability.

26 HEALTHCARE WHISTLEBLOWING

CHAPTER OVERVIEW

- ► **EXAMPLES OF CONCERNS**
- ► **RAISING CONCERNS POLICY**
- ► **RAISING CONCERNS STEPS**
- ► **EFFECTIVE PREVENTION STRATEGIES**
- ► **UNSAFE WORK ENVIRONMENT**
- ► **TIPS FOR EXECUTIVES**

EXAMPLES OF CONCERNS

- ► Abuse
- ► Indications of theft, fraud or bribery
- ► Health and safety issues and risks
- ► Abuse of power, position or authority
- ► Bullying

RAISING CONCERNS POLICY

- ► Freedom to speak up
- ► Duty of candour
- ► Honesty culture
- ► Openness

- ► Establishing a whistleblowing policy
- ► Communicating the whistleblowing policy
- ► Encouraging staff to raise concerns at an early stage
- ► Dealing with concerns promptly
- ► Reviewing the policy regularly

RAISING CONCERNS STEPS

▶ Raising informally
▶ Raising formally
▶ Escalating internally
▶ Escalating externally

▶ Internally
  • Freedom to Speak Up Guardian
  • Risk management team
  • Executive director with responsibility for whistleblowing
  • Non-executive director with responsibility for whistleblowing
▶ Externally
  • NHS Improvement
  • Care Quality Commission
  • NHS England
  • Health Education England
  • NHS Counter Fraud Authority
▶ Advice
  • Whistleblowing Helpline
  • Public Concern at Work
  • Legal representative

EFFECTIVE PREVENTION STRATEGIES

▶ Raising awareness
▶ Encouraging openness
▶ Identifying trends
▶ Leading by example
▶ Involving employees
▶ Providing training
▶ Sharing responsibility

UNSAFE WORK ENVIRONMENT

▶ Important GMC guidance
- 'Guidance to doctors working under system pressure'

▶ If a doctor believes that they are unable to maintain standards of care, the GMC urges them to flag their concerns.

▶ Raising an issue
- Senior staff member
- Medical defence organisation
- British Medical Association
- Appropriate Royal College
- General Medical Council
  - Confidential hotline

TIPS FOR EXECUTIVES

✓ Listen, consider and act on concerns.

✓ Remember: An organisational culture in which employees fear the punitive repercussions of reporting incidents poses a danger to patient safety.

✓ Avoid creating a blame culture.
✓ Shape a transparent culture encouraging issues to be raised immediately.
✓ Investigate and respond to concerns and complaints promptly.
✓ Think of whistleblowing as a way to improve the service.
✓ Provide guarantees for whistleblowing employees.

✓ 'Gagging clauses' in employment contracts are void insofar as they conflict with the protection provided by the Public Interest Disclosure Act.

✓ Be clear on how to deal with false allegations and what action will be taken if employees maliciously make a disclosure that they know to be untrue.

27 HEALTHCARE CONCERNS

CHAPTER OVERVIEW

▶ CONCERNS ABOUT DOCTORS
▶ GMC INVESTIGATION
▶ MEDICAL PRACTITIONERS TRIBUNAL SERVICE (MPTS)
▶ NATIONAL CLINICAL ASSESSMENT SERVICE (NCAS)

CONCERNS ABOUT DOCTORS

▶ Important GMC guidance
- 'A guide for doctors reported to the GMC'
- 'A guide for health professionals on how to report a doctor to the GMC'
- 'How to complain about a doctor'
- 'Raising and acting on concerns about patient safety'

▶ Most concerns about doctors will be handled locally.
▶ The GMC should be informed if there is evidence that suggests the doctor may not be fit to practise.
▶ Doctors who are reported to the GMC should
- Seek legal advice
  - Medical defence organisation
  - Specialist solicitor
  - British Medical Association
- Seek emotional support
  - Doctor Support Service

GMC INVESTIGATION

▶ Investigators
- Medical case examiner
- Non-medical case examiner
- Investigation Committee

▶ Outcome
- Closing the case
- Issuing a warning
- Agreeing undertakings to address a problem
- Referring the case to the MPTS

▶ The challenge is the tension between medical accountability and no blame.

MEDICAL PRACTITIONERS TRIBUNAL SERVICE (MPTS)

▶ Is an important statutory committee of the General Medical Council

▶ Reports to the parliament and the GMC for the delivery of their objectives

▶ Deals in hearings with doctors whose fitness to practise is called into question

▶ Has the power to impose sanctions against the doctor's registration

▶ Forms of tribunals
- During an investigation: Interim Orders Tribunal
- After an investigation: Medical Practitioners Tribunal

▶ Members of tribunals
- Both medical panellists and non-medical panellists
- Legal Assessor or Legally Qualified Chair

▶ Decisions about a doctor's fitness to practise, measured against relevant professional standards set by the GMC

▶ Outcome of a hearing
- Fitness to practise not impaired
  - Taking no action
  - Issuing a warning

- Fitness to practise impaired
  - Placing conditions on the doctor's registration
  - Suspending the doctor from the register
  - Removing the doctor from the register

▶ A doctor may appeal to the High Court or Court of Session against a decision by a medical practitioners tribunal.

▶ The Professional Standards Authority has the power to refer the decision to the High Court or Court of Session if it considers that a decision made by a medical practitioners tribunal is unduly lenient.

NATIONAL CLINICAL ASSESSMENT SERVICE (NCAS)

▶ Expert advice to healthcare organisations on the management and resolution of concerns about doctors
  - Concerns relating to knowledge and skills, health, behaviour and context of practice
    - Management of Healthcare Professional Alert Notices (HPANs)

▶ Action plans
  - Remediation action plans
  - Return to work action plans
  - Professional development action plans

28 HEALTHCARE LITIGATION

CHAPTER OVERVIEW

- ► **CLAIMS PROCEDURE**
- ► **CLAIMS PREVENTION**
- ► **TIPS FOR CLAIMS PREVENTION**
- ► **NHS RESOLUTION**

CLAIMS PROCEDURE

- ► Legal team
- ► Defence organisation
- ► Documentation of the case
- ► Statement on the allegations

CLAIMS PREVENTION

- ► High quality staff
- ► Education and training
- ► Risk management programmes
- ► Policies and procedures
- ► Accurate medical records

TIPS FOR CLAIMS PREVENTION

- ✓ Familiarise yourself with all relevant legislation, regulation, policies and procedures and how they relate to your practice.

✓ Ensure that national policies are implemented in your organisation.

✓ Take account of the NHS Constitution in all your decisions.

✓ Support high care quality.
✓ Use guidelines and protocols.
✓ Monitor team members' compliance.

NHS RESOLUTION

▶ Handles negligence claims against NHS bodies

▶ Delivers fair resolution
▶ Learns from harm
  • Operates a risk management programme to raise standards and reduce incidents
▶ Monitors human rights law
▶ Coordinates equal pay claims

29 HEALTHCARE INFORMATION

CHAPTER OVERVIEW

▶ **INFORMATION LEGISLATION**
▶ **INFORMATION GUIDANCE**
▶ **INFORMATION GOVERNANCE**
▶ **INFORMATION ACCESSIBILITY**
▶ **INFORMATION CHANNELS**
▶ **INFORMATION CULTURE**
▶ **INFORMATION FREEDOM**
▶ **INFORMATION CONFIDENTIALITY**
▶ **INFORMATION MANAGEMENT**
▶ **INFORMATION FILING**
▶ **INFORMATION DISPOSAL**
▶ **TIPS FOR INFORMATION MANAGEMENT**

INFORMATION LEGISLATION

▶ Data Protection Act
▶ Human Rights Act
▶ Equality Act
▶ Freedom of Information Act
▶ Public Interest Disclosure Act

INFORMATION GUIDANCE

▶ General Medical Council
  • 'Confidentiality – Good practice in handling patient information'
▶ Caldicott Committee principles

INFORMATION GOVERNANCE

▶ Requirements
  • Systems and processes which comply with legislation and guidance
▶ Aspects
  • Responsibilities
  • Obligations
  • Data protection
  • Information security
  • Confidentiality
  • Privacy
▶ Authority
  • Information Commissioner's Office

▶ Information governance should not be a barrier to healthcare progress.

INFORMATION ACCESSIBILITY

▶ Accessible Information Standard

INFORMATION CHANNELS

▶ Listening
▶ Speaking
▶ Writing
▶ Phoning
▶ Meeting
▶ Networking
▶ Negotiating
▶ Presenting
▶ Teamworking

INFORMATION CULTURE

▶ An excellent information culture is at the heart of a successful health service.

INFORMATION FREEDOM

▶ Emails are open to Freedom of Information requests.

INFORMATION CONFIDENTIALITY

▶ Data protection principles
  • Fairly and lawfully processed
  • Only for the purpose for which it was obtained
  • Adequate and relevant
  • Processed in accordance with the data subject's rights
  • Accurate and current
  • Only for the timeframe for which it is needed
  • Safely and securely kept

▶ Caldicott principles
  • Justify the purpose(s).
  • Do not use patient identifiable information unless it is necessary.
  • Use the minimum necessary patient identifiable information.
  • Access to patient identifiable information should be on a strict need-to-know basis.
  • Everyone with access to patient identifiable information should be aware of their responsibilities.
  • Understand and comply with the law.
  • The duty to share information can be as important as the duty to protect patient confidentiality.
▶ Caldicott guardian
  • Person with a responsibility to ensure patient data is kept secure
    ▪ 'The conscience of the organisation'

▶ Confidentiality rules of NHS Digital
  • Rule 1: Confidential information about service users or patients should be treated confidentially and respectfully.
  • Rule 2: Members of a care team should share confidential information when it is needed for the safe and effective care of an individual.
  • Rule 3: Information that is shared for the benefit of the community should be anonymised.

- Rule 4: An individual's right to object to the sharing of confidential information about them should be respected.
- Rule 5: Organisations should put policies, procedures and systems in place to ensure the confidentiality rules are followed.

▶ Need-to-know principle: Information shared must be relevant and must be proportionate to the purpose for which it is required.

▶ Reasons for a breach of confidentiality
- Safeguarding concerns
- Suspected crime
- Misconduct
- Malpractice
- Court order
- Communicable disease

INFORMATION MANAGEMENT

▶ Hospital records need to be documented, secured, stored and disposed of appropriately.

INFORMATION FILING

▶ Purpose
- Audits
- Inspections
- Reviews
- Inquiries
▶ Format
- Physical
- Electronic
▶ Requirements
- Safe
- Usable
- Transparent
- Traceable

INFORMATION DISPOSAL

▶ Retention period for records
▶ Disposal policy for records

▶ Everything which is not 'CURB'
  • Current
  • Useful
  • Required
  • Beneficial

TIPS FOR INFORMATION MANAGEMENT

✓ Do not keep information you do not need.
✓ Do keep only information which is
  • Useful
  • Up to date
  • Required

30 HEALTHCARE IT

CHAPTER OVERVIEW

► **HEALTHCARE TRENDS WITH IT RELEVANCE**
► **HEALTHCARE IT**
► **HEALTH CLOUD**
► **BIG DATA**
► **ARTIFICIAL INTELLIGENCE**
► **MACHINE LEARNING**
► **DEEP LEARNING**
► **IMAGING TRENDS WITH IT RELEVANCE**
► **TOTALLY DIGITAL RADIOLOGY DEPARTMENT**
► **ROLE OF RADIOLOGISTS**
► **IMAGING IT**
► **TIPS ON IT**

HEALTHCARE TRENDS WITH IT RELEVANCE

► Integrated healthcare
► Electronic medical records
► Personal health records
► Digital radiology department
► Digital ward rounds
► International cooperation

► Increasing budgetary pressure
► Increasing performance pressure
► Explosive growth in imaging data
► No tolerance for systems downtime

▶ Staff shortage problems
▶ Data security problems

▶ IT needs to link patients, healthcare providers and databases.
▶ IT needs to be fast, customer friendly and personalised.
▶ IT needs to improve integration, data access and workflow.

HEALTHCARE IT

▶ Medical knowledge must be actionable knowledge.

▶ IT lays the foundation for knowledge.
▶ IT is an enabler for progress in medicine.
▶ IT changes the provision of healthcare.

▶ Healthcare IT needs to provide the relevant medical information for
  • Presymptomatic care
  • Prolonged wellness

▶ Healthcare IT should be
  • Precise
  • Practical
  • Permanent
  • Performant

▶ Healthcare IT should provide
  • Relevant information
  • Significant information
  • Meaningful information
  • Purposeful information

▶ Healthcare IT should guarantee
  • Real-life data
  • Accessibility for everyone

- Connectivity with everyone
- Strict confidentiality

▶ E-connectivity and M-health improve patient safety, clinical effectiveness and patient experience.
  - They allow clinical professionals to spend their time on their core competence: diagnosing and treating patients.
▶ E-connectivity and M-health overcome professional boundaries, care divides and organisational boundaries.

▶ E-connectivity and M-health
  - E-referrals
  - E-scheduling
  - E-visits
  - E-tests
  - E-guidelines
  - E-portals
  - E-prescriptions
  - E-consulting
  - E-care
  - E-monitoring
  - E-records
    ▪ Electronic Medical Record (EMR)
    ▪ Personal Health Record (PHR)

▶ Professional-to-professional telehealth
▶ Patient-to-professional telehealth

▶ Healthcare IT should improve both workflow and thoughtflow.

▶ Success factors of healthcare IT
  - Integration
  - Simplification
  - Automation
  - Acceleration

▶ Success factors of digital strategies
  - Technological infrastructure
  - Change management
  - Organisational development
  - User friendliness
  - Data sharing
  - Learning programmes
  - Information governance
  - Sophisticated leadership

▶ Three levels of data sharing
  - Accessible
    ▪ Online data
  - Usable
    ▪ Easily discoverable and well documented data
  - Useful
    ▪ Curated and comparable data across time and place

▶ IT employees as data scientists
  - Mining data
  - Exploiting information
  - Enabling business
  - Monitoring performance

▶ Present IT era
  - Health cloud
  - Mobile technologies
  - Social technologies
  - Big data

▶ Future IT era
  - Digital revolution
  - Cognitive computing

| Health cloud
Mobile technologies
Social technologies
Big data | | Digital revolution
Cognitive computing |

HEALTH CLOUD

▶ Is a scalable, connected and secure platform
▶ Manages the volume, velocity and variety of data
▶ Improves the clinical, operational and financial outcomes

Health cloud				
Shared data	Shared applications	Shared information	Shared expertise	Shared workflow

▶ Telemedicine
▶ Teleradiology
▶ Teleconsultation

BIG DATA

▶ Definition
  • Volume
  • Velocity
  • Variety
  • Veracity
  • Value

▶ Application
  • Input analysis
  • Output analysis
  • Health information

- Health education
- Individual health analytics
- Public health monitoring
- Medical decision support
- Knowledge transfer
- Information networks
- Personalised medicine
- Scientific forecasting

▶ Relevance
- Big data as the most important resource of future medicine

▶ Governance
- Data protection
- Informational self-determination
  - 'Right to privacy'
- IT safety

ARTIFICIAL INTELLIGENCE

▶ Drivers of artificial intelligence in medicine
- Standardisation
- Quantification
- Diagnostic accuracy
- Patient safety
- Productivity
- Efficiency

▶ Value of artificial intelligence in medicine
- Decision support
  - Assistive tools to augment, quantify and stratify the available information
- Treatment improvement

▶ Value of artificial intelligence in business
- Managing staff
- Forecasting demand
- Guiding strategic decisions
- Reducing routine work
- Streamlining supply chains
- Improving customer experience
- Optimising marketing
- Personalising products
  - Leaner, cleverer and swifter organisations

▶ Artificial intelligence
- Machine learning
- Robotics, vision, speech
- Natural language processing
- Planning, scheduling, optimisation
- Expert systems

MACHINE LEARNING

▶ Machine learning
- Deep learning
- Reinforcement learning

DEEP LEARNING

▶ Deep learning
- Artificial neural networks

IMAGING TRENDS WITH IT RELEVANCE

▶ Increasing role of imaging
▶ Increasing complexity of imaging
▶ Increasing risk of litigation

▶ Radiologist: Reporting and accounting on the front end
▶ IT: Security and governance on the back end
  ● IT as a safety net for the radiologist

▶ IT needs to provide a seamless experience for the radiologist.

▶ Paramount trends
  ● Higher speed of imaging
  ● Higher degree of user friendliness
  ● Higher degree of personalisation

▶ Improved applications
  ● Visualisation of images
  ● Automation of image analysis
  ● Quantification of image characteristics
  ● Classification of findings

▶ Radiology reports
  ● Combination of text, images, measurements, graphs and metadata with added value for the referring doctor

TOTALLY DIGITAL RADIOLOGY DEPARTMENT

▶ HIS
▶ RIS
▶ PACS
▶ Cloud

▶ Patient referral
▶ Examination schedule
▶ Patient registration
▶ Image acquisition

- ▶ Image reporting
- ▶ Speech recognition
- ▶ Report distribution
- ▶ Business intelligence

- ▶ Speech recognition
- ▶ Standard texts
- ▶ Text macros
- ▶ Fill-in fields
- ▶ Predefined values
- ▶ Measurement tools
- ▶ Voice commands

ROLE OF RADIOLOGISTS

- ▶ Standardised workflow
- ▶ Pay for performance
- ▶ Pay for quality
- ▶ Flexible working hours
- ▶ Mobile working

- ▶ The radiologist should educate the clinician about requesting imaging wisely and using reports intelligently.
- ▶ The clinician should educate the radiologist about clinical decision making and effective patient care.

IMAGING IT

Patient referral ▸ Image acquisition ▸ Radiology report ▸ Multidisciplinary meetings

▶ All images and all reports should be available in the digital system for access wherever required during the care chain.

▶ Improving staff productivity
▶ Increasing patient throughput
▶ Ensuring complete transparency
▶ Supporting management decisions

▶ Mobile devices
▶ Smartphones, tablets
▶ Webinars, online conferences, apps, social media, blogs
▶ Internet, wikis
▶ Cloud services

▶ Online communities

▶ Value based healthcare
  • Manages patient referral, image acquisition, radiology report and multidisciplinary meetings
  • Focuses on outcome, quality and costs
  • Is typically manageable, actionable and measurable
  • Ensures efficient pathways, timely diagnoses, continuous care and patient empowerment

▶ Effective IT tools for value based healthcare
  • Online appointment scheduling
    ▪ Automatic confirmation
    ▪ Automatic reminders
    ▪ Patient information
    ▪ Consent form
  • Duplicate examination warnings
  • Dose management tools
  • Incident reporting solutions
  • Online chat platforms

- Mobile radiology functionalities
- Data sharing opportunities
- Structured reporting functions
  - Image integration
  - Data integration
  - Actionable information
  - Critical alerts

▶ Evaluation of value
  - Waiting time for examination?
  - Proportion of justified indications?
  - Room and examination time?
  - Staff and material costs?
  - Examinations below dose threshold?
  - Frequency of adverse events?
  - Turnaround time for reports?
  - Percentage of addenda reports?
  - Number of secondary findings?
  - Satisfaction of referring clinicians?

TIPS ON IT

✓ You must have high technical skills.
  - Rely on yourself, not on others.

✓ Develop excellent computer literacy skills.

✓ Keep up with all advances, and in particular with artificial intelligence.

31 HEALTHCARE CHALLENGES

CHAPTER OVERVIEW

- ► HEALTHCARE CHALLENGES
- ► HEALTHCARE RATIONING
- ► NHS CHALLENGES
- ► HOT TOPICS
- ► CHALLENGES FOR TRUSTS
- ► CHALLENGES FOR HOSPITALS
- ► CHALLENGES FOR LEADERS
- ► CHALLENGES FOR MANAGERS
- ► ACTION FIELDS

HEALTHCARE CHALLENGES

- ► Ageing population
- ► Growing population
- ► Sicker population
- ► Growing demands
- ► Competing demands
- ► Financial pressures
- ► Medical advancements
- ► Rising expectations
- ► Recruitment issues
- ► Workforce disenchantment

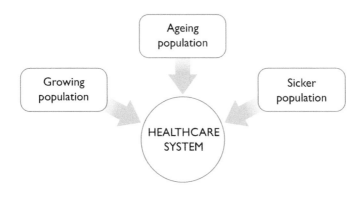

▶ Demand outpacing resources

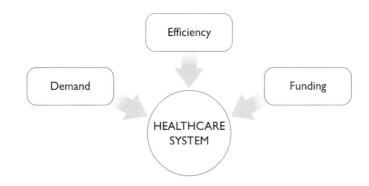

▶ Complexity
▶ Change
▶ Capability

▶ Recruitment problems
▶ Staff morale
▶ Budget cuts
▶ Pay restraints

HEALTHCARE RATIONING

▶ Rationale
  • Infinite demand versus finite resources

125

▶ Forms
- Deflection
- Delay
- Denial
- Deterrence
- Dilution

▶ QALY
- Quality adjusted life year
  - Patient's quantity of life plus patient's quality of life
  - Resource allocation in view of economic effectiveness of treatment

NHS CHALLENGES

▶ Objectives of government mandate
- Objective 1: Through better commissioning, improve local and national health outcomes, particularly by addressing poor outcomes and inequalities
- Objective 2: To help create the safest, highest quality health and social care service
- Objective 3: To balance the NHS budget and improve efficiency and productivity
- Objective 4: To lead a step change in the NHS in preventing ill health and supporting people to live better lives
- Objective 5: To maintain and improve performance against core standards
- Objective 6: To improve out-of-hospital care
- Objective 7: To support research, innovation and growth

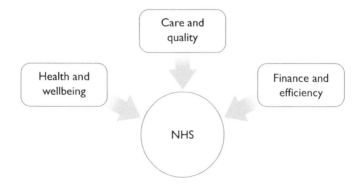

▶ Boundaries between political, managerial and clinical interests

▶ Regulatory burden
▶ Administrative burden
▶ Bureaucratic burden

▶ Too many regulatory bodies
▶ NHS too vertically structured
▶ Too many reporting requirements

▶ Lack of a single vision for the whole NHS
▶ Lack of a single communication strategy for the whole NHS
▶ Lack of a single manual for the whole NHS

HOT TOPICS

▶ Unacceptable variation in standards
▶ Urgent and emergency care
▶ New models of care
▶ Waiting times targets
▶ Seven day services
▶ Scrutiny of treatments

CHALLENGES FOR TRUSTS

▶ Effective recruitment of staff and consistent standards
▶ Best possible health outcome in the most cost effective way
▶ Data demands of regulators and oversight bodies

CHALLENGES FOR HOSPITALS

▶ Inadequate staffing
▶ Fragmentation of structures

▶ Lack of integration
▶ Failings in strategic planning
▶ Crisis of personal accountability
▶ Hygiene problems

CHALLENGES FOR LEADERS

▶ Managing competing priorities, capacity and safety imperatives, especially at times of overcrowding
▶ Addressing the impact of stress, burnout, depression and anxiety on staff
▶ Providing strategic leadership, guidance and clear advice, especially for employees in need

CHALLENGES FOR MANAGERS

▶ Public and demanding environment
▶ Difficult choices and decisions
▶ The interests of individual patients versus the interests of other people, e.g. other patients, staff, whole community, etc.
▶ Clinical and managerial priorities
▶ National and local requirements

ACTION FIELDS

▶ Long-term planning
▶ Long-term funding solutions
▶ Long-term strategy

▶ Improving leadership
▶ Supporting management
▶ Redesigning services
▶ Integrating care
▶ Reducing bureaucracy
▶ Improving performance

- ▶ Better procurement
- ▶ Better office support
- ▶ Better healthcare IT systems
- ▶ Better estate management
- ▶ Better integration

- ▶ Finding and keeping the right people with the right skills

- ▶ Community participation
- ▶ Community involvement
- ▶ Public consultations
- ▶ Public say

- ▶ Helping people manage their own health
- ▶ Designing healthcare services around the users

- ▶ Improving prevention
- ▶ Managing avoidable demand
- ▶ Reducing unwarranted variation
- ▶ Offering choice

32 HEALTHCARE TRANSFORMATION

CHAPTER OVERVIEW

▶ POLICIES
  - HEALTHCARE POLICIES
  - TARGETS AND THE NHS
  - FUNDING AND THE NHS
  - PROCUREMENT AND THE NHS
  - DRUGS AND THE NHS

▶ STRATEGIES
  - HEALTHCARE STRATEGIES
  - FIVE YEAR FORWARD VIEW
  - RADICAL UPGRADE IN PUBLIC HEALTH
  - EMPOWERMENT OF PATIENTS
  - ENGAGEMENT OF COMMUNITIES
  - NHS AS A SOCIAL MOVEMENT
  - MODELS OF CARE
  - WAYS TO SUCCESS
  - OBJECTIVE 1 FOR A HEALTHCARE ORGANISATION
  - OBJECTIVE 2 FOR A HEALTHCARE ORGANISATION
  - OBJECTIVE 3 FOR A HEALTHCARE ORGANISATION
  - OBJECTIVE 4 FOR A HEALTHCARE ORGANISATION
  - OBJECTIVE 5 FOR A HEALTHCARE ORGANISATION

▶ MANAGEMENT
  - CHANGE MANAGEMENT
    - CHANGE MANAGEMENT
  - LEAN MANAGEMENT
    - LEAN MANAGEMENT

► REORGANISATION
- HEALTHCARE SYSTEM
  - SUSTAINABILITY AND TRANSFORMATION PARTNERSHIPS (STPS)
  - INTEGRATED CARE SYSTEMS (ICSS)
  - ACCOUNTABLE CARE ORGANISATIONS (ACOS)
  - POPULATION HEALTH SYSTEM (PHS)
  - VANGUARDS
- HEALTHCARE SERVICES
  - REORGANISING HOSPITALS
  - INCREASING COMPETITIVENESS
  - BECOMING BIGGER
  - MODEL HOSPITAL
► PRIVATISATION
- HEALTHCARE PRIVATISATION
► INNOVATION
- INNOVATION STRATEGY
- INNOVATION DEGREES
- INNOVATION CULTURE

32.1. POLICIES

HEALTHCARE POLICIES

► A national debate about healthcare provision makes sense.

► Health policy should be determined by medical needs.

► Health politicians should plan for the long term.

► Healthcare executives need to understand the national context of healthcare operations.
- Wider health and social care economy
- Structure and governance arrangements
- Key roles
- Markets
- Commissioning

- Key interfaces
- Politicians and civil servants
- Political thinking and national policy making

▶ Setting political targets in healthcare
  - Scoping
  - Gathering data
  - Pitching
▶ Using political targets in healthcare
  - Monitoring
  - Providing feedback
  - Reviewing

TARGETS AND THE NHS

▶ Local control may lead to different standards in different areas.
▶ The NHS should be a truly national health service again.
  - All treatments should be available in all areas.
  - Outcomes should be the same in all areas.
▶ A seven-day-a-week NHS with excellent service provision throughout all seven days is warranted.
▶ GP surgeries need to have appointment slots in the evenings and at weekends.

FUNDING AND THE NHS

▶ Funding gaps can be bridged by reducing costs, increasing revenue or restricting services.
▶ The NHS cannot fund all new developments in healthcare.
▶ A contribution for GP and hospital visits should be considered.
▶ Foreign visitors should be charged for using NHS services.
▶ The number of regulators, authorities and officials in the NHS should be reduced.

PROCUREMENT AND THE NHS

▶ The NHS has a massive global purchasing power.
▶ Procurement procedures and price bargaining should be improved.

DRUGS AND THE NHS

▶ Drug licensing should be determined by clinical usefulness.
▶ The prescription system should reward healthy lifestyles and personal responsibility.
▶ Generic rather than branded drugs should be prescribed.

32.2. STRATEGIES

HEALTHCARE STRATEGIES

▶ As expectations increase, performance will decrease: The pre-eminent challenge is to square the unsquareable circle.

▶ Where there are challenges, there are also opportunities. It is about moving from surviving to thriving.

▶ Healthcare markets are crowded to some extent, with multiple providers chasing the same patients.
▶ Healthcare business is a matter of gaps and niches, the challenge of differentiation.
▶ Unique services and better quality offer the prospect of enduring difference and sustained profitability.

▶ Market leaders are early movers, because they are faster, or later entrants, because they are superior.
▶ A healthcare organisation stands out when its positive differences from the competing organisations are crystal clear.

▶ A healthcare organisation has a competitive advantage when it is either first or better.
▶ The quintessence of strategy is choosing what to do – and what not to do.

▶ Healthcare organisations can create a distinctive, appealing and successful brand, just like any other business.

- ► Systems and structures of healthcare organisations must be balanced with flexibility and innovation.
  - Systems and structures are for management, whereas flexibility and innovation are for leadership.
- ► Growth is the result of excellent leadership and excellent management at all levels.

- ► There is no growth without activity.
- ► Only continual progress ensures sustainable success.

- ► What today seems wrong, strange or weird may prove essential to solving tomorrow's healthcare problems.

- ► To excel, healthcare organisations need an empowered, challenged and rewarded workforce as well as a flexible, insightful and responsive leadership.
- ► This results in more individual learning and more organisational learning, which in turn leads to better care and higher productivity.

- ► Critical capabilities of successful executives in this context
  - Inclusive and compassionate leadership skills
  - Management and leadership development skills
  - System and integration leadership skills
  - Quality and performance improvement skills

- ► A healthcare organisation is a living organism.
  - It is about self-questioning.
  - It is about self-adapting.
  - It is about self-reinventing.
- ► Only this approach will ensure business survival.

- ► If a healthcare organisation is innovative, it is admired.
- ► If a healthcare organisation is safe for patients, it is safe for business.
- ► If a healthcare organisation is successful, it is irreplaceable.

FIVE YEAR FORWARD VIEW

▶ Three gaps
- Health and wellbeing gap
  - Impact: Improving health
- Care and quality gap
  - Impact: Transforming care
- Finance and efficiency gap
  - Impact: Enabling change

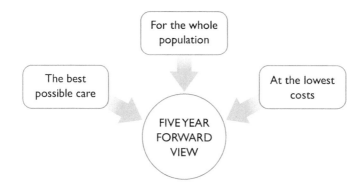

▶ Defining the right changes, the right partnerships and the right investments
▶ Dissolving the divide between
- GPs and hospitals
- Physical health and mental health
- Health care and social care
- Prevention and treatment

▶ Radical upgrade in public health
▶ Empowerment of patients
▶ Engagement of communities
▶ NHS as a social movement
▶ Models of care
▶ Ways to success

RADICAL UPGRADE IN PUBLIC HEALTH

▶ Supporting healthier behaviour
▶ Supporting local leadership on public health
▶ Supporting targeted prevention
▶ Supporting dedicated fit for work schemes
▶ Supporting workplace health

EMPOWERMENT OF PATIENTS

▶ Improving access to information
▶ Supporting people to manage their own health
▶ Increasing control over care

ENGAGEMENT OF COMMUNITIES

▶ Supporting carers
▶ Encouraging active community volunteering
▶ Cooperating with charitable organisations
▶ Managing locally

NHS AS A SOCIAL MOVEMENT

▶ Combining all initiatives and commitments in the country

MODELS OF CARE

▶ Integrating services around the patient
▶ Managing systems, i.e. networks of care, not just organisations
  • New care models
    ▪ Multispeciality Community Providers
    ▪ Primary and Acute Care Systems
    ▪ Acute Care Collaborations
    ▪ Enhanced Health in Care Homes
▶ Shifting care to community services

WAYS TO SUCCESS

▶ Joint collaboration of policymakers, regulators, commissioners and providers
▶ Joint collaboration of board, ward, patients and families

▶ Backing diverse solutions and local leadership
▶ Creating aligned national leadership
▶ Supporting a modern workforce
▶ Exploiting the information revolution
▶ Accelerating useful health innovation
▶ Driving system efficiency and productive investment

▶ Developing a patient-centred, responsive and demand-driven healthcare system
  • Competition between providers
  • Information on outcomes
  • Personal health budget
  • Choice of provider
  • Commissioning by experts

▶ Planning care with the patient, not for the patient

OBJECTIVE 1 FOR A HEALTHCARE ORGANISATION

▶ Excelling in patient safety, clinical effectiveness and patient experience

OBJECTIVE 2 FOR A HEALTHCARE ORGANISATION

▶ Ensuring the full range of services are integrated and sustainable

OBJECTIVE 3 FOR A HEALTHCARE ORGANISATION

▶ Employing the highest calibre of dedicated staff who are proud to work for the organisation

OBJECTIVE 4 FOR A HEALTHCARE ORGANISATION

▶ Working collaboratively and effectively with external partners and all stakeholders and out into the communities to ensure the best outcomes for patients at all levels

OBJECTIVE 5 FOR A HEALTHCARE ORGANISATION

▶ Being a successful organisation through maximising productivity, cost effectiveness and efficiency

32.3. MANAGEMENT

32.3.1. CHANGE MANAGEMENT

CHANGE MANAGEMENT

| Gaining insight | | Driving change | | Delivering transformation | | Achieving sustainability | | Improving value |

▶ Types of change
- Strategic change
- Operational change

▶ Types of change
- Managed change
- Evolved change
- Introduced change
- Imposed change

▶ Types of change
- Episodic change
- Radical change

▶ Steps of change
- Recognising
- Analysing
- Preparing
- Mobilising
- Communicating
- Implementing
- Evaluating
- Sustaining

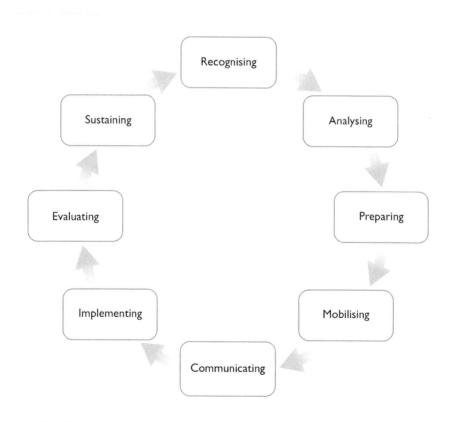

▶ Change is essential in a time of global, national and regional discontinuity, innovation and competition.

▶ If an organisation does not change, it cannot improve.

▶ Change, in the first place, is an opportunity, not a threat.

▶ Even small changes add up to something much better, as long as they are not imposed, unnecessary or mindless.

▶ Change management means managing change.
- A learning organisation is key to achieving a competitive advantage.

▶ Change management involves all staff.

▶ Change is exciting when somebody is doing it.
▶ Change is threatening when it is being done to somebody.

▶ Change management starts with me.
▶ Change management advances from 'me' to 'we'.
▶ Change management is everyone's responsibility.

▶ Change management needs to be fresh in thinking and uncompromising about quality.

▶ Change management needs to encompass the whole organisation – it is not only a top-down process.

▶ Change requires a galvanising vision and strategy.
▶ Change requires interpersonal skills.
▶ Change requires great judgement.
▶ Change requires a positive energy and empathy.

► Change requires communication.
► Change requires commitment.
► Change requires activity.
► Change requires visibility.

► Talking to staff is important. Listening to staff is even more important.
  ● Change management needs to be sensitive.
► Informing staff is important. Involving staff is even more important.
  ● Change management needs to be inclusive.

► Staff support change when they have a hand in shaping it.

► Communication approaches for change management
  ● Focus on communication strategy
    ▪ Communication objectives
    ▪ Communication tactics
    ▪ Key messages
    ▪ Communication audiences
    ▪ Communication channels
  ● Focus on priority audiences
    ▪ Opinion leaders
    ▪ Change champions
    ▪ Key stakeholders
    ▪ Known innovators
    ▪ Early adopters

► Key focus of the communication strategy
  ● Engaging people
  ● Paying attention to the vocal sceptics
  ● Sustaining interest

▶ Key enablers of the communication strategy
- Steering groups
- Advisory groups
- Lobbying groups
- Action groups

▶ Key audiences of the communication strategy
- People with interest, enthusiasm and influence
  - Board representatives
  - Staff representatives
  - Patient representatives

▶ Key questions of the communication strategy
- What?
- Why?
- When?
- Who?
- How?

▶ Key messages of the communication strategy
- Scenarios
- Probabilities
- Perspectives
- Evidence
- Data
- Examples

▶ Key attributes of the communication strategy
- Simple
- Strong
- Targeted
- Open
- Honest
- Continuous

► Staff at the heart of change
- Unlocking ambition
- Harnessing energy
- Encouraging activity
- Spreading ideas

► Staff as the agents of change

► Factors creating a sense of change
- Patient safety
- Political imperative
- Potential litigation
- Financial saving
- Process efficiency

► Factors creating a resistance to change
- Lack of education
- Lack of communication
- Lack of motivation
- Lack of participation
- Lack of involvement
- Lack of empowerment
- Lack of facilitation
- Lack of support
- Lack of recognition
- Lack of reward

► An innovative change culture requires a no blame culture.
- No blame cultures embrace the possibility of errors.
- No blame cultures value and incentivise honesty and transparency.
- No blame cultures encourage the reporting of incidents.
  - Fear is an enemy of change.
  - An innovative change culture means aiming high without fear of falling.
  - Trust is a promotor of change.

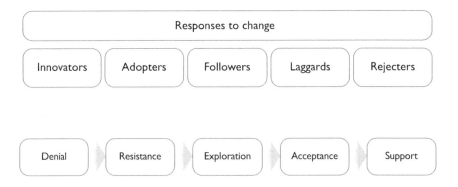

Responses to change

| Innovators | Adopters | Followers | Laggards | Rejecters |

Denial → Resistance → Exploration → Acceptance → Support

► Fundamental dimensions of change management
- Context
- Content
- Organisation
- SWOT
- Stakeholder
- Process
- Cycle

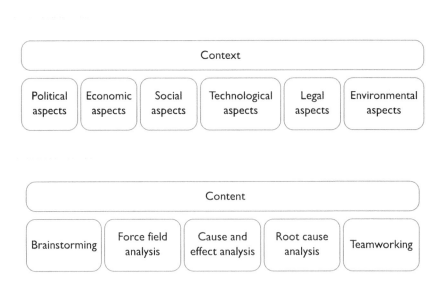

Context

| Political aspects | Economic aspects | Social aspects | Technological aspects | Legal aspects | Environmental aspects |

Content

| Brainstorming | Force field analysis | Cause and effect analysis | Root cause analysis | Teamworking |

Organisation					
System	Structure	Strategy	Style	Staff	Skills

SWOT			
Strengths (internal factors)	Weaknesses (internal factors)	Opportunities (external factors)	Threats (external factors)

Stakeholder			
Winners inside the organisation	Losers inside the organisation	Winners outside the organisation	Losers outside the organisation

Process					
Communicating openly	Consulting effectively	Engaging actively	Knowing the legal duties	Understanding the emotional journey	Demonstrating a strong leadership

Cycle			
Plan	Do	Check	Act

▶ Basic principles of change management
- Building on strengths
- Addressing weaknesses
- Exploiting opportunities
- Dealing with threats

▶ Basic approaches to change management
- Change as an exception versus change as the norm
- Incremental change versus radical change
- Change as a process versus change as an upheaval

▶ Key enablers of change management
- Committed and respected leadership
- Change culture
- Engaged staff
- Enabling environment
- Adequate resources
- Exact data
- Excellent communication
- Team skills
- Flawless execution and implementation

▶ Key disablers of change management
- No recognition of the need for change
- No motivation for change
- No headspace for change
- No capability for change
- No support from the board for change

▶ It is easier to change structures and processes than attitudes and mindsets.

▶ Evaluation of change management in healthcare
- Internal
- External
  - Simple, up to date and relevant to ensure practical usefulness

▶ Evaluation of change management in healthcare
- Continuity
- Sustainability
  - Short term action to ensure long term transformation

▶ Essential contents of the evaluation report
- Executive summary
- Introduction
- Background
- Method
- Findings
- Discussion
- Recommendations
- Lessons learned

32.3.2. LEAN MANAGEMENT

LEAN MANAGEMENT

▶ Success factors of a lean culture
- Committed leadership
- Sense of urgency
- Lean improvement method
- Alignment of expectations
- Shared vision

▶ Radical elimination of waste in patient care
- Waste is defined as interventions which do not add value.
▶ Radical implementation of efficiency in patient flow

- ▶ The organisational culture has a strong impact on business behaviour.
- ▶ The organisational culture comprises attitudes, approaches, feelings, beliefs, values, standards, routines, rituals – the way things are done.
- ▶ The organisational culture is an important determinant of business success.

- ▶ The organisational culture should be geared towards excellence and execution.

- ▶ Examples of lean approaches in healthcare
  - ● Care bundles
    - ▪ Collection of evidence based interventions
    - ▪ Means to ensure that the application of all interventions is consistent for all patients and at all times
    - ▪ Tool for health outcome improvement
  - ● Just in time
  - ● No more bottlenecks
  - ● Walk-in walk-out services
  - ● Show and go
  - ● One stop shop
  - ● Patient empowerment

32.4. REORGANISATION

32.4.1. HEALTHCARE SYSTEM

SUSTAINABILITY AND TRANSFORMATION PARTNERSHIPS (STPS)

- ▶ Main vehicle for redesigning services
- ▶ Main vehicle for transforming health and care services in line with the NHS Five Year Forward View
- ▶ Main vehicle for sustaining services

- ▶ Geographical division of England into STP areas
  - ● Areas agreed between NHS trusts, clinical commissioning groups and local authorities

▶ Plan implementation through leaders of each area
- Improving care quality
- Promoting population health
- Working across organisational borders
- Developing new care models
- Restoring financial balance
- Maintaining financial stability

▶ Key themes common to all partnerships
- Workforce
- Prevention
- New care models
- Urgent care
- Primary care
- Secondary care
  - Reconfiguration
  - Consolidation
  - Cooperation
- Community care
- Mental health
- Consultation and engagement
- Funding
- Commissioning

INTEGRATED CARE SYSTEMS (ICSS)

▶ An integrated care system is an evolved version of a sustainability and transformation partnership.
- An ICS brings together a number of providers who take responsibility for the quality and cost of care for a defined population within an agreed budget.

▶ Collaborative working between primary, hospital, community and social care services

149

ACCOUNTABLE CARE ORGANISATIONS (ACOS)

▶ Integrated care systems may lead to the establishment of an accountable care organisation.

POPULATION HEALTH SYSTEM (PHS)

▶ The key theme is full integration.

▶ STPs, ICSs and ACOs point to the emergence of population health systems, which seek to integrate care and to improve the broader health and the wellbeing of the local population.

▶ Dimensions of population health systems
  • Big data
  • Population analysis
  • Digital health
  • Artificial intelligence
  • Public health
  • Comprehensive prevention
  • Case management
  • Self care
  • Healthcare delivery
  • Healthcare costs
  • Patient engagement
  • Patient empowerment

VANGUARDS

▶ Vanguards have been introduced as part of the NHS Five Year Forward View.

▶ Aims
  • Developing new care models
    ▪ Better patient care
    ▪ Better service access

- Generating a blueprint for the future of the NHS
- Redesigning the healthcare system

▶ Values
- Clinical engagement
- Patient involvement
- Local ownership
- National support

▶ Integrated primary and acute care system (PACS) vanguards
▶ Multispeciality community provider (MCP) vanguards

32.4.2. HEALTHCARE SERVICES

REORGANISING HOSPITALS

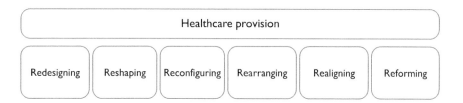

Healthcare provision

| Redesigning | Reshaping | Reconfiguring | Rearranging | Realigning | Reforming |

▶ Reorganisation process
- Involving and consulting the staff from the outset of the process
- Listening to suggestions
- Acknowledging the input
- Accepting solutions born out of necessity
- Showing that the impossible is possible
- Creating and developing a multi site care environment and team culture

▶ Reorganisation process
- Generating collective competence
    ▪ Giving everyone an equal voice
- Developing collective ownership

▶ Optimising health services along care pathways
▶ Shifting healthcare from an acute towards a community setting
▶ Centralising acute services across all sites
▶ Establishing differentiated but complementary roles for the hospitals involved

▶ Concentrating expertise
▶ Maximising quality and outcomes
▶ Making better use of existing resources
▶ Minimising duplication and cost
▶ Increasing competitiveness

INCREASING COMPETITIVENESS

▶ Becoming bigger
- Alliances
- Chains
- Joint ventures
- Multilateral cooperations
    ▪ Expansion of services
    ▪ Economies of scale
    ▪ Strengthened bargaining positions
    ▪ Unique selling propositions
- Mergers
- Acquisitions
▶ Becoming better
- Talent management
- Staff training
- Process optimisation
- Innovation culture

▶ Becoming closer
- Referral base
- Community relations
- Outpatient networks
- Telemedicine services

BECOMING BIGGER

▶ Advantages of becoming bigger
- Providing strategic leadership
- Centralising appropriate functions
- Achieving greater economies of scale and skill
- Driving sustainable transformation
- Standardising practice effectively

▶ Disadvantages of becoming bigger
- Problem: Mismatch of cultures
  - Example: 'A' with a formal and hierarchical culture, 'B' with an informal and democratic culture, 'AB' with a mismatching culture
- Result: Lack of synergy

MODEL HOSPITAL

▶ One source of data, benchmarks and best practice
▶ One integrated performance framework which is centred around patients, staff and finances
▶ One version of quality, efficiency and strategic perspectives

▶ Comparison of performance and productivity across organisations
- Adjusted treatment cost (ATC)
- Weighted activity unit (WAU)

▶ Benchmarking between organisations

32.5. PRIVATISATION

HEALTHCARE PRIVATISATION

▶ The private sector has always played a major role in health provision.
  • Examples are dentists, GPs, physiotherapists and pharmacies.

▶ Involvement of the private sector does not mean privatisation of the public sector.

▶ The 'public good, private bad' mindset is as wrong as the 'public bad, private good' attitude.
  • People do not care, as long as they get the services they want, where they want and when they want.
▶ Public and private sector healthcare services should operate side by side and compete with each other.

▶ Potential advantages of private healthcare
  • More competition
  • More choice
  • More capacity
  • Top specialists
  • Early treatment
  • Better quality
  • Better facilities
  • Better services

▶ Potential disadvantages of private healthcare
  • Rising inequality
  • Cherry picking
  • Decreasing level of public healthcare provision with increasing level of private healthcare provision
  • Limited cover
  • Rising costs

▶ Patients with complex conditions or increased needs are usually screened out and treated in the public sector.

32.6. INNOVATION

INNOVATION STRATEGY

▶ Elements of an innovation strategy
- Clear set of choices
- Integrated set of activities
- Based on demand, evidence and capability
- Evolving to outcomes, performance and success

▶ Development of an innovation strategy
- Company analysis
- Competence analysis
- Customer analysis
- Competitor analysis

▶ Alignment of an innovation strategy
- Definition of key milestones
- Framework for strategic initiatives
- Based on projects, plans and processes
- Evolving to quality, growth and efficiency

▶ Success of an innovation strategy
- Comprehensible strategy
- Communicable strategy
- Implementable strategy
- Executable strategy

INNOVATION DEGREES

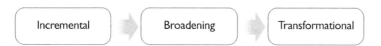

Incremental → Broadening → Transformational

INNOVATION CULTURE

▶ Components of an innovation culture
- Compassionate leadership
- Mission

- Vision
- Values
- Inspiration
- Strategy
- Systems thinking
- Cross boundary working
- Transformational change
- Empowerment
- Inclusion
- Participation
- Support
- Autonomy
- Enthusiastic teamwork

33 HEALTHCARE PERSONALISATION

CHAPTER OVERVIEW

► **HEALTHCARE PERSONALISATION**
► **RISK TAKING**
► **RELEVANT LEGISLATION**
► **ETHICAL DILEMMAS**
► **OPTIMAL OUTCOME**

HEALTHCARE PERSONALISATION

► Putting people in the centre and in control
► Fitting the service around the individual – not the individual into the service
  • The people who use the service make decisions – not the staff who deliver the service.
    ▪ Implementing Individual Service Funds
► Recognising and treating people as individuals and partners

From the 'deficit model' Looking at things a person is unable to do: Disabilities	To the 'asset model' Looking at things a person is able to do: Abilities	Health services fill in any gaps the person identifies: Personalised care

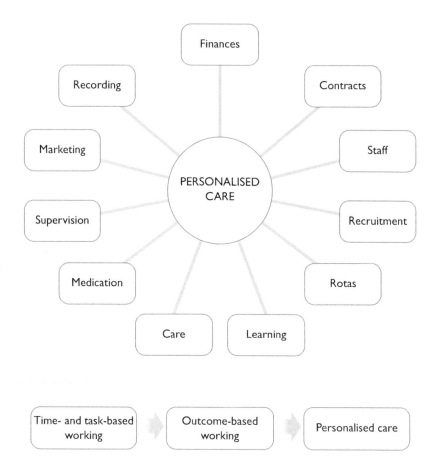

► Families, friends and the local community are important in a personalised service.

► Giving people choice, independence and control implies giving them the right to take a risk.

RISK TAKING

► Learning to live with risk
► Principles of working with risk
  • Risk identification
  • Risk assessment

- Multidisciplinary and interagency working in proportion to the risk and impact to self and others
- Decision making
- Decision recording

▶ An inevitable consequence of providing a personalised service is that staff will have to balance an approach to risk against their duty of care.

▶ There is a fundamental distinction between enabling people to choose to take a risk and putting people at risk.

RELEVANT LEGISLATION

▶ Mental Capacity Act
▶ Mental Health Act
  - Deprivation of Liberty Safeguards
▶ Human Rights Act

▶ Everyone is assumed to have capacity unless there is evidence that they do not.
▶ Any decisions made on behalf of a person who lacks capacity must be in their best interests.
  - Mental Health Assessor
  - Best Interest Assessor

ETHICAL DILEMMAS

▶ Balancing rights of individuals and duty of care
  - Finding workable agreements to appease all parties involved
    - Applying sound judgement
    - Respecting dignity and autonomy
    - Promoting equality and diversity
    - Upholding fairness and justice
    - Minimising risk and harm
    - Showing great compassion

▶ Balancing rights of individuals and duty of care
- As a rule of thumb, encouraging and supporting individual decision making
  ▪ As far as is reasonably possible
  ▪ As long as the rights of others are not infringed
  ▪ As far as is reasonably practicable

▶ Balancing rights of individuals and duty of care
- Lasting Power of Attorney
- Advance decisions
  ▪ Right of self-determination and of autonomy
- Court of Protection Deputy

OPTIMAL OUTCOME

▶ Rewards of personalised care for the patient
- Patient safety
- Patient quality of life
- Patient experience

▶ Rewards of personalised care for the organisation
- Service quality
- Improved job satisfaction
- Higher staff retention
- Reduced safeguarding concerns
- Positive feedback

34 HEALTHCARE JOBS

CHAPTER OVERVIEW

▶ PREPARATION
- SOURCES OF JOB INFORMATION
- JOB RELATED WEBSITES
- JOB POSTING WEBSITES
- SPECIALISED RECRUITMENT AGENCIES
- PROFESSIONAL MEMBERSHIP ORGANISATION
- PROFESSIONAL HEALTHCARE JOURNALS
- HEALTHCARE POLICY DATA

▶ APPLICATION
- TIPS FOR THE JOB MARKET
- TIPS FOR TAKING FULL CONTROL
- TIPS FOR GETTING GREAT JOBS
- TIPS FOR SOCIAL MEDIA PROFILES
- TIPS FOR A BRILLIANT CV
- TIPS FOR THE COVER LETTER
- TIPS FOR THE APPLICATION FORM
- TIPS FOR A SUCCESSFUL INTERVIEW
- TIPS FOR THE PERFECT JOB

34.1. PREPARATION

SOURCES OF JOB INFORMATION

▶ Job related websites
▶ Job posting websites
▶ Specialised recruitment agencies

- ▶ Professional membership associations
- ▶ Professional healthcare journals
- ▶ Healthcare policy data

JOB RELATED WEBSITES

- ▶ NHS Leadership Academy
  - http://www.leadershipacademy.nhs.uk
- ▶ NHS Confederation
  - http://www.nhsconfed.org
- ▶ NHS Employers
  - http://www.nhsemployers.org
- ▶ NHS Health Education England
  - https://www.healthcareers.nhs.uk

JOB POSTING WEBSITES

- ▶ Job search
- ▶ Careers advice
- ▶ Uploading a CV
- ▶ Jobs by email
- ▶ Recruiter search
- ▶ Headhunting database

- ▶ British Medical Journal
  - https://jobs.bmj.com
- ▶ Health Service Journal
  - http://www.hsjjobs.com
- ▶ NHS
  - https://www.jobs.nhs.uk
- ▶ Find a job
  - https://www.gov.uk/jobsearch
- ▶ Jobs.ac.uk
  - http://www.jobs.ac.uk
- ▶ Academic Positions
  - http://academicpositions.co.uk

▶ Doc2UK
  ● https://doc2uk.com
▶ Doctors.net.uk
  ● http://www.doctors.net.uk

SPECIALISED RECRUITMENT AGENCIES

▶ NHS Leadership Academy Executive Search
  ● http://execsearch.leadershipacademy.nhs.uk
▶ Recruitment and Employment Confederation
  ● https://www.rec.uk.com
▶ Hunter Healthcare
  ● http://www.hunter-healthcare.com
▶ Michael Page
  ● https://www.michaelpage.co.uk
▶ Perrett Laver
  ● http://www.perrettlaver.com
▶ Veredus Healthcare
  ● https://www.veredus.co.uk/health

▶ Connecting the world's most influential organisations with the world's most dynamic leaders
  ● Recruiting without borders
  ● Recruiting across sectors
    ▪ Identifying the best leaders
    ▪ Engaging the best leaders
    ▪ Securing the best leaders

PROFESSIONAL MEMBERSHIP ORGANISATION

▶ Faculty of Medical Leadership and Management
  ● https://www.fmlm.ac.uk

PROFESSIONAL HEALTHCARE JOURNALS

▶ BMJ Leader
  ● http://bmjleader.bmj.com
▶ Health Service Journal
  ● http://www.hsj.co.uk
▶ National Health Executive
  ● http://www.nationalhealthexecutive.com

HEALTHCARE POLICY DATA

▶ Department of Health
  ● https://www.gov.uk/government/organisations/department-of-health-and-social-care
▶ Office for National Statistics
  ● https://www.ons.gov.uk/peoplepopulationandcommunity/healthandsocialcare
▶ NHS England
  ● https://www.england.nhs.uk

34.2. APPLICATION

TIPS FOR THE JOB MARKET

✓ Visible job market
  ● Reading job advertisements is key.
✓ Invisible job market
  ● Networking with peers is key.
    ▪ Good relationships may lead to job referrals.
    ▪ Give to get.
    ▪ Help others and they will help you.

TIPS FOR TAKING FULL CONTROL

✓ Do not leave anything to chance.
✓ Do not leave the responsibility to others.
✓ Take control of the application process.
✓ Take control of the communication with others.

✓ Steer your application to a successful outcome. Keep a firm grip on the wheel.

✓ It is you who should ring the recruiter or the employer. Do not sit down and wait for them to call you.

TIPS FOR GETTING GREAT JOBS

✓ Create job alerts.
✓ Get your name on the files of agencies. The recruitment consultant or search consultant will connect you with potential employers.
✓ Upload your CV.

✓ Approach services proactively.
✓ Ask when jobs will be coming up.
✓ Learn what they are ideally looking for.
✓ Develop productive relationships.

✓ Headhunters have a vested interest in applicants, because no placement means no fee.

TIPS FOR SOCIAL MEDIA PROFILES

✓ List your achievements, specialities and skills. Strictly focus on what is preferred, advantageous and desirable for the post.

TIPS FOR A BRILLIANT CV

✓ Your curriculum vitae is your marketing tool.
  - It is a statement of fact.
  - It is a proof of achievements.
  - It is a document of quality.

✓ Keep your CV
- Structured
- Relevant
- Accurate
- Concise
- Consistent
- Current

✓ Pay attention to
- Logical order
- Relevant keywords
- Powerful wording
- Bullet points

✓ Structure is key
- Personal details
- Current position
- Education and qualifications
- Distinctions and honours
- Career history
- Skills and experience
- Leadership experience
- Research and teaching
- Publications and presentations
- Personal interests
- Three referees

✓ Start with a summary of your key achievements on the first page.

✓ List not only your roles but also your accomplishments.

✓ Be prepared. Express your value in terms of outcomes. Be factual.

✓ Focus attention on
- Performance
- Key contributions
- Successes
- Notable achievements
  - Clinical
  - Academic
  - Managerial
  - Personal

✓ Customise your application.

✓ Match your qualifications, skills and experience to the job description, person specification and organisational values.
- Tailor your CV to the role, but always stick to the truth.

✓ Pay attention to coded text and hidden criteria in the job description.

✓ Proofread your CV carefully. Proofread it again. And then proofread it.

TIPS FOR THE COVER LETTER

✓ List the strong areas of your application in a short list of bullet points.

TIPS FOR THE APPLICATION FORM

✓ Give sufficient importance to application forms.

TIPS FOR A SUCCESSFUL INTERVIEW

✓ Getting the interview
- Be employer friendly.

- Be there to take the calls of a potential employer.
- Be easily available.

✓ Preparing for the interview
  - Organisation's website
  - Interviewer profiles
  - Possible questions from the interviewers
  - Own questions for the interviewers
  - CV memorised
  - Documents ready

✓ Preparing for the interview
  - Informal (pre-interview) visit
    ▪ Online information about the organisation
    ▪ Region, area, facilities, people, 'vibe'
    ▪ SWOT analysis of the department
  - Formal (interview) visit
  - Audiovisual presentation
  - Psychometric test

✓ How you look, speak and write reflects your upbringing, culture and values.

✓ Think smart, look smart and be smart.

✓ Take visual aids to the interview, e.g. publications, books, brochures, etc.

✓ Positive thinking is key.
✓ Feeling confident is actually being confident.
✓ Keep eye contact with the interviewers.
✓ Relax and be yourself.

✓ Early and last impressions matter.
  - 'We know one when we see one.'
✓ Early and last impressions stick.

....

✓ Your best points must come out.
✓ Take control of the interview.
✓ Get all your key messages across.

....

✓ Listen intently.
✓ Respond intelligently.
✓ Stay focused.

....

✓ Stand out from the crowd.
✓ List strengths but also examples that demonstrate these.
✓ Respond to questions thoughtfully, truthfully, concisely and completely.
✓ Stay away from your weaknesses.

....

✓ Focus on what marks you out from the others: your personality, your uniqueness, your individuality. What makes you special?

....

✓ What is the major and unique contribution to the organisation that only you can make? Specify the added value.

....

✓ Do not hide your light under a bushel.

....

✓ Emphasise the value of team effort, team play and team work in life by using 'we' and 'us' in your descriptions, rather than 'I' and 'me'. Project the image of someone who fits in.

....

✓ It is all about your strengths, motivation and fitness. Focus on the salient points. Explain clearly why these are benefits to the organisation. Finish with a strong conclusion.

✓ Stop when you have finished. Do not talk too much.

✓ Give evidence for what you say.
✓ Use your track record of success.
✓ Focus on typical work related examples.

✓ Think of ways to overcome the weaknesses in your application. A pre-emptive strike can be an effective solution. Turn the negative into the positive.

✓ Remember: Your application will be scored according to how closely you meet the selection criteria.

✓ Respectfully thank the interviewers and other staff for their time.
✓ Let them know that you enjoyed learning more about the organisation and position. Say that you are clear about the remit and challenges of the job. Reemphasise your motivation for applying.
✓ Say that you look forward to hearing from the interviewers.

TIPS FOR THE PERFECT JOB

✓ There is always a way in. But you need to be persistent.

✓ Persuasiveness and tenacity are essential tools in your quest for success and happiness.

35 HEALTHCARE EMPLOYMENT

CHAPTER OVERVIEW

- ► WORKPLACE
  - GOOD EMPLOYERS
  - WORKPLACE IMPROVEMENTS
- ► WORKFORCE
  - NHS WORKFORCE
  - WORKFORCE THEMES
  - WORKFORCE PRIORITIES
  - WORKFORCE PLANNING
  - WORKFORCE SHORTAGE
  - NHS EMPLOYERS
  - TIPS FOR EXECUTIVES
- ► RECRUITMENT
  - FILLING POSITIONS
  - HIRING STAFF
  - SELECTING STAFF
  - VALUE BASED RECRUITMENT PROCESS
  - MANAGEMENT OF STAFF SHORTAGES
  - PROFILE OF CONSULTANTS
  - JOB PLANNING FOR CONSULTANTS
  - CAREER OF CONSULTANTS
- ► TRAINING
  - HEALTH EDUCATION ENGLAND (HEE)
  - LOCAL EDUCATION AND TRAINING BOARDS (LETBS)
  - LOCAL EDUCATION PROVIDERS
  - TEACHING METHODS
  - IMPROVING TRAINING OF JUNIOR DOCTORS

▶ WELLBEING
- ASPECTS OF WELLBEING
- CHALLENGES TO WELLBEING
- WELLBEING AND PERFORMANCE
- WELLBEING AND LEADERSHIP
- WELLBEING AND MANAGEMENT
- DEFINITION OF RESILIENCE
- APPROACHES TO RESILIENCE
- ROADS TO RESILIENCE

▶ STRESS
- DEFINITION OF STRESS
- CAUSES OF STRESS
- CONSEQUENCES OF STRESS
- TIPS TO COMBAT STRESS
- DEFINITION OF BURNOUT
- CAUSES OF BURNOUT
- SIGNS OF BURNOUT
- CONSEQUENCES OF BURNOUT
- STRATEGIES TO PREVENT BURNOUT
- DOCTORS IN DIFFICULTY

▶ LAW
- DISCLAIMER
- SOURCES OF EMPLOYMENT LAW
- TRIBUNAL AND COURT SYSTEM
- CONTRACT OF EMPLOYMENT
- TERMINATION OF EMPLOYMENT
- DISMISSAL
- DISCRIMINATION

▶ DISCIPLINE
- DISCLAIMER
- ADVISORY, CONCILIATION AND ARBITRATION SERVICE (ACAS)
- DISCIPLINING STAFF
- TIPS FOR EXECUTIVES

35.1. WORKPLACE

GOOD EMPLOYERS

▶ Performance indicators of good employers
- Employee satisfaction
- Role satisfaction
- Staff recommendation
- Absence rate
- Training and development
- Management and leadership
- Work environment
- Benefit packages
- Corporate culture
- Corporate communications

WORKPLACE IMPROVEMENTS

▶ Action fields for workplace improvements
- Staff engagement framework
- Staff innovation panels
- Staff resilience training
- Childcare provision
- Equality and diversity measures
- Training and development plans
- Coaching and mentoring programmes
- Question and answer sessions
- Positive environment
- Personal health counselling
- Flexible working options
- Job share arrangements

35.2. WORKFORCE

NHS WORKFORCE

▶ British NHS as the largest employer in the UK and in Europe
- 8500 separate organisations
- 1.7 million staff
- 350 different careers

WORKFORCE THEMES

▶ Key themes
- Well-trained workforce, well-motivated workforce
- Effective recruitment, selection, retention and remuneration
- Staff productivity, staff efficiency
  - Building top leadership at all levels

WORKFORCE PRIORITIES

▶ Top priority
- Preparing the workforce to do new things in new ways, under new conditions, with new horizons

WORKFORCE PLANNING

▶ Health Education England (HEE)
▶ Local Education and Training Boards (LETBs)
▶ Centre for Workforce Intelligence (CFWI)
- Supports senior leaders in driving workforce planning
- Provides workforce intelligence to the healthcare system
- Provides best practice to improve workforce efficiency
▶ Social Partnership Forum (SPF)
- NHS Employers, NHS England, Department of Health, Health Education England, NHS trade unions

WORKFORCE SHORTAGE

▶ Addressing the workforce shortage in healthcare
  - Increasing supply
  - Creating a supportive work environment
  - Improving multi-disciplinary and multi-professional working
  - Retaining staff

NHS EMPLOYERS

▶ NHS Employers represents employing organisations in the health service on workforce issues.

▶ Priority areas
  - Staff pay and negotiations
  - Recruitment and workforce planning
  - Healthy and productive workplaces
  - Employment policy and practice

TIPS FOR EXECUTIVES

✓ Reduce reliance on medical locums.
✓ Engage in the optimal planning, deployment and design of the existing workforce.
✓ Work supportively with neighbouring trusts.

✓ Also reduce reliance on medical locums by improving working conditions, flexible shift patterns and rota management.

35.3. RECRUITMENT

FILLING POSITIONS

▶ Advertising
▶ Approaching
▶ Networking
▶ Headhunting

HIRING STAFF

- ▶ Job description
- ▶ Person specification
- ▶ Information pack
- ▶ Application form
- ▶ Equality and diversity monitoring form
- ▶ Job offer letter
- ▶ Written Statement of Terms and Conditions of Employment
- ▶ Checklists
  - Staff recruitment checklist
  - Pre-employment checklist
  - Job induction checklist

- ▶ Important NHS Employers guidance
  - 'Employment checks document cross reference tool'
    - Identity checks
    - Right to work checks
    - Criminal record checks

SELECTING STAFF

- ▶ Structured interview
  - Open questions
  - Closed questions
  - Capability questions
  - Probing questions
- ▶ Psychometric test
- ▶ Work simulation
- ▶ Assessment centre

- ▶ Initially, staff should be selected for attitude.
- ▶ Then, staff should be trained for skill.

- ▶ Past performance is the best predictor of future performance.

VALUE BASED RECRUITMENT PROCESS

▶ Recruits people who embrace the workplace values
▶ Incorporates values in
  • Job advertisements
  • Job descriptions
  • Person specifications
  • Shortlisting criteria
  • Interview questions
  • Interview scoring

MANAGEMENT OF STAFF SHORTAGES

▶ Increasing training numbers
▶ Devising recruitment incentives
▶ Employing locum staff
  • Locum agencies
  • Recruitment consultants
▶ Recruiting from abroad
▶ Improving employee orientation
  • Flexible working
  • Job sharing
  • Unpaid leave
  • Pension schemes
  • Sabbaticals
  • Secondments
  • Occupational health
  • Wellbeing programmes
  • Recognition schemes
  • Childcare facilities

▶ Recruitment premium
▶ Relocation packages
▶ Pastoral support
▶ Induction programmes

- ▶ Talent management
- ▶ Social events
- ▶ Staff benefits
- ▶ Retention premium

PROFILE OF CONSULTANTS

- ▶ Providing specialist clinical expertise
- ▶ Bearing ultimate clinical responsibility
- ▶ Acting as patients' advocates
- ▶ Conducting research
- ▶ Leading innovation
- ▶ Assuring quality
- ▶ Practising management
- ▶ Providing leadership
- ▶ Providing junior doctors' training
- ▶ Offering specialist clinical advice
- ▶ Developing hospital trusts' policies

JOB PLANNING FOR CONSULTANTS

- ▶ Professional obligation
- ▶ Contractual obligation

- ▶ Annual job planning meeting
- ▶ Medical job plan consistency committee
- ▶ Electronic job planning system

- ▶ Programmed activities
  - Direct clinical care
  - Supporting professional activities
    - Management
    - Research
    - Education
    - Governance

- Audit
- Appraisal
  - Additional responsibilities
    - Audit lead
    - Department lead
    - Clinical Director
    - Medical Director
  - External duties
    - General Medical Council
    - Medical Royal Colleges
    - Care Quality Commission
    - Department of Health
- On call
  - Frequency
  - Category
- Private practice

CAREER OF CONSULTANTS

- Junior consultant
  - Emphasis on clinical work
- Senior consultant
  - Emphasis on management, leadership, teaching, research

35.4. TRAINING

HEALTH EDUCATION ENGLAND (HEE)

- Ensuring that the workforce of today and tomorrow has the right numbers, skills, values and behaviours, at the right time and in the right place
  - Planning and developing the workforce
  - Promoting quality education and training

LOCAL EDUCATION AND TRAINING BOARDS (LETBS)

- Committees of Health Education England
- Development of local NHS staff

LOCAL EDUCATION PROVIDERS

▶ Education and training of staff

TEACHING METHODS

▶ Lecture
▶ Demonstration
▶ Problem based learning
▶ Seminar
▶ Tutorial

IMPROVING TRAINING OF JUNIOR DOCTORS

▶ Enhanced training flexibility
  • Time out from clinical duties
  • Less than full time training
▶ Improved rota designs
▶ Upgraded study budgets
▶ Extension of training periods in the same department
▶ Integration in the team structure of the respective department
▶ Standardisation of the annual review of competence progression
▶ Upgraded feedback systems
▶ Improved mentoring opportunities
▶ Enhanced teaching facilities

35.5. WELLBEING

ASPECTS OF WELLBEING

▶ Physical
▶ Emotional
▶ Intellectual
▶ Spiritual
▶ Social

▶ Cultural
▶ Economic
▶ Environmental

CHALLENGES TO WELLBEING

▶ Workload
▶ Pressure
▶ Overwhelm
▶ Uncertainty
▶ Change
▶ Complaints
▶ Criticism
▶ Lack of communication
▶ Lack of feedback
▶ Lack of support
▶ Lack of control
▶ Solitude
▶ Disputes
▶ Conflict
▶ Bullying
▶ Harassment
▶ Discrimination
▶ Litigation

WELLBEING AND PERFORMANCE

▶ Link between wellbeing of employees and
  • Patient outcome
  • Patient experience
  • Staff absence
  • Staff turnover
  • Individual productivity
  • Organisational productivity

WELLBEING AND LEADERSHIP

▶ Leadership aspects
- Having a wellbeing vision
- Understanding the wellbeing needs
- Identifying the wellbeing activities
- Creating a wellbeing strategy
- Appointing a wellbeing lead
- Training the line managers
- Communicating the wellbeing strategy
- Implementing the wellbeing strategy
- Taking a targeted approach
  - Focusing on behaviour change techniques
  - Focusing on encouraging staff to take personal responsibility
  - Focusing on available support services
- Evaluating the wellbeing objectives
- Acting upon the findings

WELLBEING AND MANAGEMENT

▶ Management aspects
- Counselling
- Mentoring
- Taking organisational measures
- Arranging professional help
- Mediating
- Conciliating

DEFINITION OF RESILIENCE

▶ Ability to manage and overcome adverse events without experiencing stress

APPROACHES TO RESILIENCE

▶ Problem focused
▶ Emotion focused
▶ Solution focused

ROADS TO RESILIENCE

▶ Colleagues
▶ Team
▶ Friends
▶ Family
▶ Purpose and vision
▶ Flexibility and adaptability
▶ Courses and workshops
▶ Mentoring and coaching
▶ Self esteem
▶ Personal development
▶ Organisational policies
▶ Decisive actions

35.6. STRESS

DEFINITION OF STRESS

▶ Adverse reaction to excessive demands or high pressure

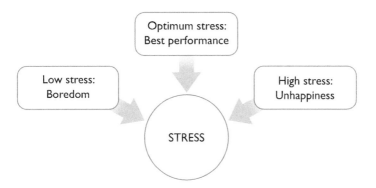

CAUSES OF STRESS

▶ Type of work
▶ Amount of work

▶ Lack of support
▶ Lack of control
▶ Quality of relationships
▶ Change of workplace

CONSEQUENCES OF STRESS

▶ Burnout
▶ Depression
▶ Anxiety
▶ Back pain
▶ Heart disease
▶ Drug dependency

TIPS TO COMBAT STRESS

✓ Disconnect.
✓ Prioritise.
✓ Refocus.
✓ Reenergise.

DEFINITION OF BURNOUT

▶ Extended response to unrelenting stress

CAUSES OF BURNOUT

▶ Work overload
▶ Role erosion
▶ Perpetual busyness
  • Race against the clock
▶ Information overload
▶ Economic uncertainties

SIGNS OF BURNOUT

▶ Apathy
▶ Cynicism
▶ Detachment
▶ Disillusionment
▶ Dissatisfaction
▶ Exhaustion
▶ Frustration
▶ Inefficacy
▶ Pessimism
▶ Tiredness

CONSEQUENCES OF BURNOUT

▶ Loss of effectiveness, balance and happiness

STRATEGIES TO PREVENT BURNOUT

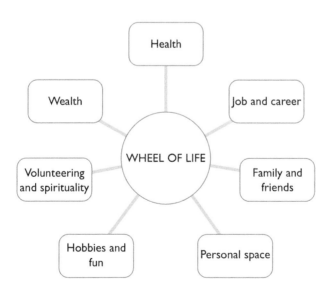

▶ Better work-life balance
- Better physical, emotional and cognitive relationship between work and home

▶ Better work-life balance
- Employees should find ways of how to meet their responsibilities.
- Employees should have autonomy over how they achieve their goals.
- The focus should only be on results and outcomes.
- The focus should not be on where and how.

▶ Better work-life balance
- Flexible working
- Reduced time
- Compressed schedules
- Time off
- Home working
- Job sharing
- Childcare assistance
- Occupational health
- Consistent approaches
- Individual solutions

▶ Better workplace atmosphere
- Sense of purpose
- Sense of togetherness
- Sense of appreciation
- Sense of gratitude
- Sense of care

▶ Better job design
- More flexible work
- More interesting work
- More challenging work
- More training opportunities

- Less boring work
- Less repetitive tasks
- Less work overload
- Less time pressure

DOCTORS IN DIFFICULTY

▶ Management of doctors in difficulty
- Patient safety comes first
- Identifying the problem
- Collecting all information
- Following organisation's guidelines
- Asking for advice
- Patient safety comes first

▶ Remember: Patient safety comes first.

35.7. LAW

DISCLAIMER

▶ The factsheets in this book are not intended as legal advice. Consult an expert on the specifics of your issue.

SOURCES OF EMPLOYMENT LAW

▶ Statute
- Parliament Act
- Statutory Instrument
▶ Case Law

TRIBUNAL AND COURT SYSTEM

▶ Employment Tribunal
▶ Employment Appeal Tribunal

▶ Court of Appeal, Civil Division
▶ Supreme Court

CONTRACT OF EMPLOYMENT

▶ Express terms
  • Terms agreed between parties
▶ Implied terms
  • On the part of the employer
    ▪ Duty to pay wages
    ▪ Duty to exercise reasonable care
    ▪ Duty to provide a grievance procedure
    ▪ Duty of mutual trust and confidence
  • On the part of the employee
    ▪ Duty of obedience
    ▪ Duty to adapt
    ▪ Duty to exercise care
    ▪ Duty of fidelity or good faith
▶ Imposed terms
  • Terms imposed by statute

TERMINATION OF EMPLOYMENT

▶ Termination by way of contract
▶ Termination in breach of contract
▶ Termination by methods external to the contract

DISMISSAL

▶ Reason for the dismissal
  • Potentially fair
    ▪ Capability or qualifications
    ▪ Conduct
    ▪ Redundancy
    ▪ Contravention of statutes
  • Automatically unfair
    ▪ Pregnancy

- Union membership
- Union representative
- Whistleblowing

▶ Fairness of the dismissal
- Band of reasonable responses
  - 'Could a reasonable employer have done what was done?'
- Procedural fairness
  - 'ACAS Code of Practice'

▶ Remedies for unfair dismissal
- Reinstatement
- Re-engagement
- Compensation

DISCRIMINATION

▶ Protected equality characteristics
- Age
- Disability
- Gender reassignment
- Marriage and civil partnership
- Pregnancy and maternity
- Race
- Religion or belief
- Sex
- Sexual orientation

35.8. DISCIPLINE

DISCLAIMER

▶ The factsheets in this book are not intended as legal advice. Consult an expert on the specifics of your issue.

ADVISORY, CONCILIATION AND ARBITRATION SERVICE (ACAS)

▶ Supports good relationships between employers and employees which underpin business success

▶ Governed by an independent council, including representatives of employer and employee organisations and employment experts

▶ Provides information, advice, training, conciliation and other services for employers and employees to help prevent or resolve workplace problems

▶ Priority areas
  • Workplace relations
  • Employment law
▶ Useful templates
  • Checklists
  • Forms
  • Letters
  • Questionnaires
  • Tips
  • Tools

▶ ACAS Code of Practice on Discipline and Grievance Procedures
  • Investigation
  • Disciplinary meeting
  • Disciplinary action
  • Appeal

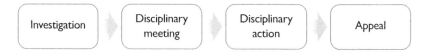

DISCIPLINING STAFF

▶ Managers should seek advice from Human Resources, ACAS or legal advisers to ensure they comply with the relevant procedures and legislation. Procedures can be contractual and not following the procedures could lead to a breach of contract.

▶ Disciplinary action
  - First stage
    - Improvement note for unsatisfactory performance
    - First written warning
  - Second stage
    - Final written warning
  - Third stage
    - Transfer
    - Demotion
    - Loss of pay
    - Suspension
    - Dismissal

▶ Referring information about a dismissal or resignation as a result of serious concerns
  - Disclosure and Barring Service (DBS)
  - Local safeguarding team
  - Professional regulatory body
  - Healthcare Professional Alert Notices (HPANs)

TIPS FOR EXECUTIVES

✓ Deal promptly.
✓ Act consistently.
✓ Carry out investigations.
✓ Inform the employee about the allegations.
✓ Allow the employee to present his/her case.
✓ Explain the right to be accompanied.
✓ Keep brief notes.
✓ Be objective.
✓ Be fair.

✓ Always keep clear records, because if it is not written down, it did not happen.

36 HEALTHCARE DIVERSITY

CHAPTER OVERVIEW

▶ STAFF
- HEALTHCARE DIVERSITY
- CULTURAL INTELLIGENCE
- MANAGING MULTICULTURAL TEAMS
- TIPS FOR MANAGING DIVERSITY

▶ LANGUAGE
- LANGUAGE ISSUES
- ADVANTAGES OF WORKING IN ONE'S OWN LANGUAGE
- ADVANTAGES OF WORKING IN A FOREIGN LANGUAGE
- TIPS FOR WORKING IN A FOREIGN LANGUAGE

36.1. STAFF

HEALTHCARE DIVERSITY

▶ Different staff backgrounds
- Ethnic
- Religious
- Cultural

▶ Different staff languages
▶ Different staff attitudes
▶ Different staff mindsets
▶ Different staff habits
▶ Different staff gestures

▶ Employees' diverse perspectives result in better patient care provided that the team members think independently, but together.

- The more diverse the team, the more representative the ideas.

▶ Differences between people make a team think creatively.
▶ Differences between people enhance performance by combining complementary strengths.
▶ Differences between people make a team pull together.

▶ Diversity means more momentum, more potential, more creativity, more innovation, more flexibility, more productivity – and more fun.

▶ Diverse, cross-departmental, cross-functional and collaborative wins.
▶ Similar, single-handed, single-sided and siloed loses.

▶ Uniformity is death.

CULTURAL INTELLIGENCE

▶ Ability to understand unfamiliar contexts and then to adjust

▶ Three dimensions
- Cognitive: Head
- Physical: Body
- Emotional: Heart

▶ First stage
- Perceptiveness
- Adaptability
▶ Second stage
- Head, body and heart in line

MANAGING MULTICULTURAL TEAMS

▶ Common themes
  • Command of language
  • Style of conversation
  • Approach to work
  • Attitude towards hierarchy
  • Sense of belonging

▶ Main objectives
  • Increasing cultural awareness
  • Increasing cultural curiosity
  • Increasing cultural empathy
  • Increasing team identity
  • Increasing team spirit

▶ Main objectives
  • Reducing communication barriers
  • Reducing emotional tensions
  • Reducing interpersonal frictions
  • Reducing unjustified prejudices
  • Reducing team conflicts

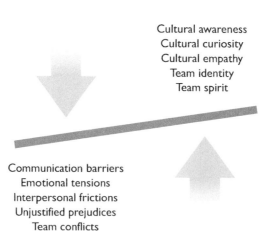

Cultural awareness
Cultural curiosity
Cultural empathy
Team identity
Team spirit

Communication barriers
Emotional tensions
Interpersonal frictions
Unjustified prejudices
Team conflicts

▶ Four steps for managing a multicultural team
- ● First step: Adaptation strategy
  - ▪ Encouraging employees
- ● Second step: Managerial intervention
  - ▪ Guiding employees
- ● Third step: Structural intervention
  - ▪ Reassigning employees
- ● Fourth step: Exit strategy
  - ▪ Removing employees

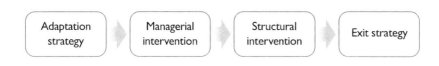

▶ Integration values cultural differences.
▶ Integration overcomes assimilation ('We are all the same') and differentiation ('We are all very different').
▶ Integration promotes equal opportunities.

▶ Healthcare executives of today should have international experience, multilingual skills, contextual understanding, semantic awareness – and the ability to switch easily between different cultures.

▶ International teams should be familiar with the norms and behaviours of multiple cultures – they need cross-cultural abilities.

▶ The best strategy is to acknowledge the cultural gaps – and then to develop a common understanding.

TIPS FOR MANAGING DIVERSITY

✓ Leave your comfort zone and see what else is out there.

✓ Value diversity.

✓ Practise an inclusive leadership style.

✓ Encourage an open discussion about diversity.

✓ Eliminate all forms of discrimination.

✓ Progress equality.

✓ Treat all employees fairly.

- Provide transparent information.
- Avoid personal bias.
- Apply policies consistently.
- Reward people equitably.

✓ Challenge power imbalances.

✓ Do not ostracise employees.

✓ Increase personal contact.

✓ Focus on people's desire to look good to other people.

✓ Promote social accountability.

✓ Expect full participation from everyone.

✓ Expect high performance standards from everyone.

✓ Expect personal development from everyone.

✓ Create an ethical culture.

✓ Make your organisation a great place to work.

✓ Deliver cumulative performance improvements.

✓ Treat organisational values and conduct codes as absolutes.

✓ Basically, it is all about common courtesy: Treat others the way you want to be treated.

36.2. LANGUAGE

LANGUAGE ISSUES

▶ English is the lingua franca.
▶ Non-native English speakers are vastly outnumbering native English speakers.
▶ Standard English has many variations.

▶ Lack of language fluency can lead to underestimation of competence.
▶ Difficulties in communicating knowledge can lead to perceptions of incompetence.

▶ Working in one's own language: Obvious advantages
▶ Working in a foreign language: Subtle advantages

ADVANTAGES OF WORKING IN ONE'S OWN LANGUAGE

▶ Arguing fluently
▶ Making a point subtly
▶ Lightening the mood with a joke
▶ Holding the conversation floor
▶ Feeling safe

ADVANTAGES OF WORKING IN A FOREIGN LANGUAGE

▶ Arguing less emotionally
▶ Speaking slowly to choose the right words
▶ Asking for clarification to buy valuable time or to distract from problems
▶ Thinking twice to reach a wise decision
▶ Behaving with modesty

TIPS FOR WORKING IN A FOREIGN LANGUAGE

✓ Be aware of your language command and communication habits.

✓ Ask native speakers to slow down, to avoid jargon and to clarify content.

....

✓ Aim to speak the foreign language fluently and idiomatically in order to get ready for nuanced discussions.

....

✓ Structure your thinking.
✓ Practise common scenarios.
✓ Do not focus on grammar or accent but on content and rhetoric.
✓ Perfect your body language.
✓ Laugh at your mistakes.

....

✓ If at first you do not succeed, try again.

....

✓ When in Rome, do as the Romans do.

37 HEALTHCARE COMMUNICATION

CHAPTER OVERVIEW

- ▶ COMMUNICATION DEFINITION
- ▶ COMMUNICATION TYPES
- ▶ COMMUNICATION ASPECTS
- ▶ COMMUNICATION QUALITY
- ▶ COMMUNICATION METHODS
- ▶ COMMUNICATION CHANNELS
- ▶ COMMUNICATION LEVELS
- ▶ COMMUNICATION PRINCIPLES
- ▶ COMMUNICATION BARRIERS
- ▶ COMMUNICATION EFFECTIVENESS
- ▶ TIPS FOR EFFECTIVE COMMUNICATION

COMMUNICATION DEFINITION

- ▶ Transfer of meaning from a sender to a receiver

- ▶ Encoding and decoding messages

COMMUNICATION TYPES

- ▶ Advising
- ▶ Assessing
- ▶ Counselling
- ▶ Criticising
- ▶ Informing
- ▶ Instructing

▶ Observing
▶ Welcoming

COMMUNICATION ASPECTS

▶ What (message)?
▶ Why (purpose)?
▶ Who (audience)?
▶ When (timing)?
▶ Where (place)?

COMMUNICATION QUALITY

▶ Content
▶ Clarity
▶ Format
▶ Style
▶ Spelling

COMMUNICATION METHODS

▶ Verbal
▶ Written
▶ Electronic
▶ Visual
▶ Nonverbal

COMMUNICATION CHANNELS

▶ Talks
▶ Meetings
▶ Speeches
▶ Roadshows
▶ Emails
▶ Letters

► Intranet
► Social media
► Smartphone apps
► Staff handbooks
► Payslip leaflets
► Internet
► Notes
► Noticeboards
► Posters
► Newsletters
► Reports
► Records

COMMUNICATION LEVELS

► Intrapersonal
► Interpersonal
► Organisational
► Public

COMMUNICATION PRINCIPLES

► Continuous
► Dynamic
► Circular
► Irreversible
► Complex

COMMUNICATION BARRIERS

► External
  • Environmental aspects
  • Cultural aspects
► Internal
  • Self awareness
  • Self reflection

- ▶ Background
- ▶ Education
- ▶ Experience
- ▶ Feelings
- ▶ Prejudices
- ▶ Stereotypes
- ▶ Language
- ▶ Medium
- ▶ Situation

COMMUNICATION EFFECTIVENESS

▶ Communication is a critical skill for executives. Excellent communication can turn listeners into followers. Communication is a key priority for organisations.

▶ Communication provides information, creates alignment and executes strategy.

▶ Clarity and brevity are the success factors of effective communication.

▶ People generally only remember
  - 10% of what they read
  - 20% of what they hear
  - 30% of what they see

▶ Questions play an important role in communication.

▶ Impact of questions
  - Questions lead from information to knowledge.
  - Questions lead from uncertainty to confidence.
  - Questions lead from mental fog to clear focus.
  - Questions lead from poor processing to wise execution.
  - Questions lead from darkness to light.
  - Questions lead from present to future.

► Impact of questions
  - Questions connect people.
  - Questions develop ideas.
  - Questions unlock wisdom.
  - Questions open doors.
  - Questions solve problems.
  - Questions transform organisations.

TIPS FOR EFFECTIVE COMMUNICATION

✓ Listen actively.
  - Acknowledge.
  - Reflect.
  - Restate.
  - Paraphrase.
  - Clarify.
  - Summarise.
✓ Neutralise feelings.
✓ Take a non-judgemental approach.
  - Accept the other person.
  - Show unconditional positive regard for the other person and be non-directive.
    ▪ Preoccupation obstructs communication.
  - Value the other person.
✓ Be sincere.
✓ Be empathetic.
  - Relax.
  - Uncross arms and legs.
  - Lean slightly towards the other person.
  - Maintain good eye contact.
  - Focus.

✓ Control your core message.
  - Objective, contents, impact
✓ Control your voice.
  - Volume, pitch, tone

✓ Control your body language.
  • Posture, gestures, expression

✓ Prepare thoroughly.
✓ Communicate clearly.
✓ Reinforce systematically.
  • Repeat important information in written form.
  • Use iterations and analogies.
  • Ask your colleagues for appropriate feedback.

✓ Successful communication is an ongoing process.

✓ Verify that your message is being understood.
✓ Verify that your message is perceived in the way you intended.
✓ Verify that your message is acted upon.

✓ Speak and look. – Make a deliberate pause. – Listen and contemplate.

✓ Hold the pause: Silence gives emphasis, gravitas and authority.

✓ A pause and matching body language reinforce your words.

✓ Speak less. Master your language. Choose your words wisely – they may come back. Speak slowly. Keep eye contact.

✓ Do not digress. Do not waffle. Keep the conversation to the point. Avoid unnecessary anecdotes. Avoid excessive pleasantries.

✓ Convey authenticity, authority, credibility and conviction.

✓ Say what you mean.
✓ Mean what you say.

....

✓ Ask questions.
✓ Show interest.
✓ Encourage openness.
✓ Value dissenting opinions.
✓ Be upfront.
✓ Be forthright.
✓ Be positive.

....

✓ Leverage the 'why' question, the 'what if' question and the 'how' question.

....

✓ Get the message. Read between the lines. Read the nonverbal cues. Decode the truth.

....

✓ Bear in mind that communication is the basis for real understanding between different parties.

....

✓ Ignorance leads to rumours, false assumptions and speculation.

....

✓ Avoid preconceived ideas.
✓ Keep an open mind.
✓ Confront your biases.

....

✓ Beware of selective hearing and wishful thinking.

....

✓ Address people by name.

....

✓ Use polite and diplomatic forms of expression
  • I think ...
  • I feel ...

- I believe …
- Shouldn't we …
- Couldn't you …
- Wouldn't it …
- I'm afraid …
- I regret …
- I'm sorry …

✓ Remember the power of a smile.

✓ Never let the communication break down.
- Problems within an organisation can often be traced back to a lack of communication.

✓ Always keep everyone in the loop.

38 HEALTHCARE MEETINGS

CHAPTER OVERVIEW

► **PURPOSE OF MEETINGS**
► **GUIDELINES FOR MEETINGS**
► **CHAIRING MEETINGS**
► **MEETING MINUTES**
► **TIPS FOR EFFECTIVE MEETINGS**

PURPOSE OF MEETINGS

► Informing
► Brainstorming
► Producing
► Deciding
► Networking
► Promoting
► Celebrating

GUIDELINES FOR MEETINGS

► Planning
► Preparing
► Participating
► Pursuing

► Starting on time
► Beginning with clear objectives
► Encouraging active discussion

▶ Discouraging irrelevant contributions

▶ Pressing for results

▶ Summarising key points

▶ Taking good meeting notes

▶ Finishing on time

CHAIRING MEETINGS

▶ Key responsibilities
- Before the meeting
  - Planning the agenda
  - Identifying which agenda items are for information, discussion or decision
  - Preparing the documents
- During the meeting
  - Communicating
  - Controlling
  - Coaxing
  - Comparing
  - Clarifying
- After the meeting
  - Summarising the decisions
  - Agreeing on dates for future meetings and the next agenda
  - Circulating the minutes

▶ Success factors
- Keeping control
- Knowing the aims
- Listening to others
- Making all members feel valued and new members feel welcome
- Striving for consensus
- Selling the benefits
- Keeping calm

MEETING MINUTES

▶ Headings

▶ Subheadings

▶ Clear structure
▶ Short sentences
▶ No abbreviations
▶ Lists
▶ Graphics

TIPS FOR EFFECTIVE MEETINGS

✓ Ask yourself
  • Do I really need to schedule a meeting?
  • Do I really need to attend a meeting?

✓ Leave committees if your presence is not essential.

✓ Meetings must have a clear objective. Make sure you meet that objective.

✓ Start meetings on time. Never wait for anyone.

✓ Meetings should be as short as possible. This is in the interest of everyone.

✓ Prepare the ground by talking to key participants before the meeting.

✓ Identify powerful allies of your proposals and brief them in advance, if possible.
✓ Meet possible adversaries of your proposals and convert them in advance, if possible.

✓ Avoid confrontations at large meetings.

✓ Chair the meeting with firmness and politeness.
✓ Treat the participants with consideration and courtesy.

✓ Ensure reasonable discussion.

✓ Clarify incomprehensible contributions.

✓ Summarise key points.

✓ Eliminate cross-talk.

✓ Oppose hierarchical attitudes.

✓ Oppose individual dominance.

✓ Oppose undue influence.

✓ Oppose social conformity.

✓ Rotate seating assignments.

✓ Ensure that all participants have their moment in the sun.

✓ Remember that poor meetings are time wasters.
  - What is the outcome of the meeting?
  - Are the decisions being converted into actions?
  - What is the return on time invested?

✓ Conclude the meeting by specifying who will do what and by when.

✓ Provide action steps.

✓ Pay attention to 'cabinet responsibility', i.e. commitment to agreement after the meeting.

39 HEALTHCARE PRESENTATIONS

CHAPTER OVERVIEW

▶ **PURPOSE OF PRESENTATIONS**
▶ **GUIDELINES FOR PRESENTATIONS**
▶ **TIPS FOR EFFECTIVE PRESENTATIONS**

PURPOSE OF PRESENTATIONS

▶ Informing the audience

▶ Changing the mindset of the audience
▶ Changing the behaviour of the audience

▶ Shifting the present state of the audience to the desired state
   • Generating fresh thoughts
   • Generating fresh feelings
   • Generating fresh actions

GUIDELINES FOR PRESENTATIONS

▶ Knowing the purpose
▶ Knowing the audience
▶ Knowing the venue
▶ Knowing the contents
   • Speaking notes with key points

TIPS FOR EFFECTIVE PRESENTATIONS

✓ Use presentations to make a connection with people.
  - Presentations are not for the speaker, but for the audience.
✓ Use presentations to make an impact on people.

✓ Know the knowledge level of your audience and move on from there.

✓ Place special emphasis on gatekeepers, opinion leaders and key decision makers.

✓ Limit the number of topics.
✓ Limit the number of slides.
  - Limit the bullets.
  - Limit the text.
  - Limit the details.
  - Use expressive headlines.
  - Use visual aids.
  - Use specific examples.
✓ Limit the number of statements.

✓ Prepare.
✓ Rehearse.
✓ Practise.

✓ Be alert.
✓ Stand straight.
✓ Breathe regularly.
✓ Be positive.

✓ Head up: mentally, physically and emotionally.

✓ Acknowledge the audience.
✓ Break the ice.
✓ Make eye contact.
✓ Ensure maximum comfort.
✓ Thank the audience.

✓ Start your presentation with inclusive statements.
  • Alternatively, start your presentation with an icebreaker.
✓ Continue your presentation with leading statements.

✓ Inclusive statements followed by leading statements guarantee a powerful opening.

✓ Speak with energy.
✓ Speak with conviction.
✓ Speak clearly.
✓ Speak succinctly.

✓ Use words that resonate.
✓ Use pauses for emphasis.

✓ Enunciate properly.

✓ Control your voice.
  • Modify volume, pitch, tone and speed.

✓ Energise.
✓ Engage the heart and mind.
✓ Emotionalise.

✓ Start strong and end even stronger.

✓ Be sure to pause frequently so that the audience can catch up and make sense of your statements.

✓ Finish each thought before you move on.

✓ Capture the essence, vigorously and persuasively. Visual support clarifies, explains and reinforces the spoken word. Speak and show, simply and clearly.

✓ Humanise, personalise and concretise your theme.

✓ Understand the power of a story.
✓ Persuade through the art of storytelling.
✓ Dramatise your topic.
✓ Emotionalise your message.

✓ Plan the segues. A presentation must flow logically and naturally from slide to slide. Keep it rolling.

✓ End with a mighty crescendo.
✓ End with easy-to-remember take-home messages.
  • Capture the essence.
  • Send a signal.
  • Call to action.
✓ End in a timely fashion.

✓ Make your presentation memorable.
✓ Deliver content.
✓ Deliver impact.
✓ Convey clarity.

✓ Convey passion.

✓ Close on a high.

. . . .

✓ Answering questions after the presentation
- Acknowledge.
- Paraphrase.
- Answer.
- Explain.
- Check.
- Debrief.

. . . .

✓ Anticipate answers to questions which participants might ask you after the presentation.

. . . .

✓ Prepare robust answers and compelling evidence to adversarial questioning or hostile feedback.

40 HEALTHCARE NEGOTIATIONS

CHAPTER OVERVIEW

► GUIDELINES FOR NEGOTIATIONS
► STYLES OF NEGOTIATIONS
► OUTCOMES OF NEGOTIATIONS
► BARGAINING IN NEGOTIATIONS
► TIPS FOR EFFECTIVE NEGOTIATIONS

GUIDELINES FOR NEGOTIATIONS

► Knowing the negotiation subject
  • Facts
  • Objectives
  • Arguments
► Knowing the negotiation process
  • Preparing
  • Opening
  • Bargaining
  • Closing
► Knowing the negotiation strategy
  • Ideal
  • Target
  • Minimum

STYLES OF NEGOTIATIONS

► Competing: I win – you lose
► Collaborating: I win – you win

► Compromising: I win/lose some – you win/lose some
► Avoiding: I lose – you lose
► Accommodating: I lose – you win

OUTCOMES OF NEGOTIATIONS

► No way
► My way
► Your way
► Half way
► New way

BARGAINING IN NEGOTIATIONS

► Integrative bargaining is preferable to distributive bargaining.

► Integrative bargaining creates win-win solutions and builds long-term relationships.

TIPS FOR EFFECTIVE NEGOTIATIONS

✓ Prepare your 'must-haves', your 'ideals' and your 'give-aways'.
✓ Prepare your position, your requirements and your reaction.
✓ Be patient.
✓ Be empathetic.

✓ Get the best outcome you can, but be fair and play by the rules.

✓ Find common ground.
✓ Seek an agreement.
✓ Build fair consensus.

✓ Your success does not require someone else's failure.

✓ How can this agreement benefit both of us?
  - It is all about mutuality.

....

✓ Do not become impatient.
✓ Give as well as take.
✓ Do not become confrontational.

....

✓ If possible, decline a battle.
✓ If that is not possible, pick your battles.
✓ Never fight a lost battle.

....

✓ Brilliant minds cooperate – and win the day.

....

✓ Negotiations take a lot of time. But if an agreement is reached, it is reached. Do not go back on it.

....

✓ Do not talk much. Silence is golden in negotiations. Keep your powder dry.

....

✓ Make your decisions on the basis of goals and results, not on the basis of emotions and pressure.

....

✓ End positively.

41 HEALTHCARE PROJECTS

CHAPTER OVERVIEW

- ▶ PROJECT DEFINITION
- ▶ PROJECT CHARACTERISTICS
- ▶ PROJECT PHASES
- ▶ PROJECT START
- ▶ PROJECT PLAN
- ▶ PROJECT SCHEDULE
- ▶ PROJECT RISKS
- ▶ PROJECT FAILURE
- ▶ PROJECT TEAM
- ▶ PROJECT SPONSOR
- ▶ PROJECT MANAGER
- ▶ BUSINESS CASE
- ▶ TIPS FOR PROJECT MANAGERS

PROJECT DEFINITION

- ▶ Title
- ▶ Background
- ▶ Goals
- ▶ Scope
- ▶ Constraints
- ▶ Justification
- ▶ Expectations

PROJECT CHARACTERISTICS

- ▶ It must be started.

- It must have a specific goal.
- It must be managed.
- It must have a time frame.
- It must be closed.

PROJECT PHASES

- Initiation
- Definition
- Planning
- Control
- Implementation
- Review

PROJECT START

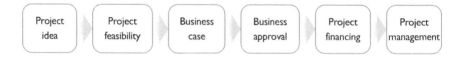

Project idea → Project feasibility → Business case → Business approval → Project financing → Project management

PROJECT PLAN

- Goals and objectives
  - Specific
  - Measurable
  - Achievable
  - Relevant
  - Timed
- Constraints and restrictions
  - Meaningfulness
  - Time
  - Budget
  - People
  - Organisation
  - Culture

- Commitment
- Compliance
- Standards
- Law

PROJECT SCHEDULE

▶ Project stages
- Time frame

PROJECT RISKS

▶ Risk sources
- Medical progress
- Business environment
- Legislative changes
- Skills shortage

▶ Risk analysis
- Risk identification
- Risk estimation
  - Risk probability
  - Risk impact
- Risk evaluation
  - Risk prioritisation
  - Risk countermeasures
- Risk recording

▶ Risk countermeasures
- Prevention
- Reduction
- Contingency
- Acceptance

▶ Risk management
- Planning
- Resourcing
- Monitoring
- Controlling

PROJECT FAILURE

▶ Main reasons for project failure
- Nebulous goals
- Changing objectives
- Unrealistic expectations
- Conflicting interests
- Poor leadership
- Ambiguous responsibilities
- Insufficient support
- Inadequate financing

PROJECT TEAM

▶ Team recruitment
▶ Team development
▶ Team meetings
▶ Skills matrix
▶ Availability matrix
▶ Productivity matrix

▶ Team recruitment
- Paramount importance

▶ Team development
- Tuckman stage 1: Forming
- Tuckman stage 2: Storming
- Tuckman stage 3: Norming
- Tuckman stage 4: Performing

▶ Team meetings
- Kick off meeting
- Informal one-to-one and face-to-face meetings
- Regular progress meetings

PROJECT SPONSOR

▶ The project sponsor confers the authority and responsibility for a project on the project manager.

PROJECT MANAGER

▶ The project manager reports the progress and outcome of the project to the project sponsor.

▶ Key skills
- Planning
- Organising
- Leading
- Controlling

▶ Key tasks
- Clarifying the goals
- Developing the plan
- Steering the project
- Managing the risks
- Communicating with stakeholders
- Motivating the team
- Measuring the progress
- Analysing the problems
- Achieving the goals

▶ Key tasks
- Evaluating the results against the plan, i.e. objectives and deliverables

▶ Project managers initiate, manage and implement change.

▶ Project managers need management knowledge, negotiation skills and common sense.

BUSINESS CASE

- ▶ Preface
- ▶ Contents
- ▶ Summary
  - Results
  - Recommendations
- ▶ Introduction
  - Strategic context
  - Evidence base
  - Scope
  - Objectives
- ▶ Analysis
  - Assumptions
  - Costs
  - Revenue
  - Benefits
  - Risks
  - Implications
- ▶ Interpretation
  - Strategic options
  - Wider impact
  - Funding
  - Implementation
- ▶ Timetable
  - Evaluation
  - Outcomes
- ▶ Conclusion
- ▶ Appendix

TIPS FOR PROJECT MANAGERS

- ✓ Believe in the project.
- ✓ Advocate for the project.
- ✓ Engage in the project.

✓ Be organised, committed and proactive.

....

✓ Early stages of a project: Build the team.
✓ Middle stages of a project: Identify and resolve any conflicts.
✓ Late stages of a project: Motivate the team.

....

✓ Notice, comment, encourage and reward. Small gestures mean the most.

....

✓ Define major operations and subsidiary tasks.
✓ Determine realistic milestones and tangible steps.

....

✓ Deal with stakeholders
   • A – Interested and powerful: Involve.
   • B – Interested but not powerful: Inform.
   • C – Powerful but not interested: Consult.
   • D – Not interested and not powerful: Monitor.

....

✓ Start your project with a structure, determination and much enthusiasm.
✓ Pursue your project with good ideas, entrepreneurial spirit and business acumen.
✓ Close your project with results, on time and within budget.

....

✓ Start small – but think big.
✓ Work hard – and follow through.

....

✓ Keep the faith.
✓ Beat the odds.

42 HEALTHCARE WORKFLOW

CHAPTER OVERVIEW

- ► **TIME MANAGEMENT**
- ► **TIPS FOR TIME MANAGEMENT**
- ► **EFFECTIVE DELEGATION**
- ► **TIPS FOR EFFECTIVE DELEGATION**
- ► **EFFECTIVE READING**
- ► **TIPS FOR EFFECTIVE READING**
- ► **EFFECTIVE WRITING**
- ► **TIPS FOR EFFECTIVE WRITING**
- ► **LIFE GOALS**
- ► **TIPS FOR LIFE GOALS**

TIME MANAGEMENT

- ► Basic principles of work organisation
  - Tracking time
  - Analysing results
  - Developing plans
  - Setting priorities
  - Reallocating time

- ► Broad categories of job duties
  - Core responsibilities
  - Administrative work
  - People management
    - ▪ Managing up
    - ▪ Managing across
    - ▪ Managing down

- Urgent matters
- Personal development

▶ Key problems of time management
  - There seems to be too much to do …
  - And there seems to be not enough time …

▶ Workplace time killers
  - Internal
    - Unorganised workspace
    - Poor delegation
    - Procrastination
    - Backlogs
    - Inefficient habits
    - Pointless routine
  - External
    - Changing priorities
    - Fire fighting
    - Distractions
    - Interruptions
    - Unplanned meetings
    - Unexpected visitors

▶ General time killers
  - Redundant processes
  - Excessive information
  - Waiting for people
  - Waiting for services
  - Technical defects
  - Unnecessary commuting

▶ Worst time killers
  - Lack of self discipline
  - Things beyond one's control
  - Demands of other people

TIPS FOR TIME MANAGEMENT

✓ Plan your day.
  • Prioritised work comes first.

✓ Plan your day.
  • Plan time for unscheduled activities.
  • Allow time for creative thinking.
  • Allow time for pondering problems.
  • Allow time for considering options.
  • Plan time for short breaks.

✓ Plan your day.
  • Group similar tasks together.
  • Set up time boxes.
  • Define realistic time limits.
  • Keep yourself on track.

✓ Prioritise your tasks.
  • A – Important and urgent: Do.
  • B – Important but not urgent: Delay.
  • C – Urgent but not important: Delegate.
  • D – Not important and not urgent: Discard.

✓ Prioritise your tasks.
  • Heed the Pareto Principle or 80/20 rule stating that the few (20%) are vital and the many (80%) are trivial.
    ▪ 20% of your efforts produce 80% of your results.

✓ Prioritise your tasks.
  • Prioritise value over volume.
  • Focus on tasks that really matter.
  • Get everything necessary done.

✓ Plan your time in order to control your time.

....

✓ Answer the key questions: What do you need to do more of? What do you need to do less of?

....

✓ An increasing workload means you need to work smarter – rather than harder, longer or faster. You can get much more done by doing much less.

....

✓ Achieve more with less energy.
✓ Done is better than perfect.

....

✓ Focus on top outcomes, not on office time.

....

✓ Get balance back.
  • It is all about productivity, not about longer hours, a workaholic culture or depressing treadmills.
✓ Live your life.

....

✓ And there is more good news: If you believe in something, if you believe in what you are doing, if you believe in yourself – it will not feel like work.

....

✓ Always channel your energy intelligently.
✓ Do not spend time on inconsequential matters.
✓ Make sure you are perfectly organised, dedicated, focused and ruthlessly efficient.
✓ Optimise your thought patterns and work habits.
✓ Streamline everything and save time.

....

✓ Do not procrastinate.
  • Procrastination is the thief of time and the inhibitor of success.
✓ Do not postpone.

....

✓ Think in terms of days and weeks, not months and years.

....

✓ Set yourself a deadline.

✓ Never put off until tomorrow what you can do today.

✓ Get on with it.

✓ Design your office consciously and keep a clear desk for a clear brain.

✓ Be helpful, but do not be too reactive to the demands of other people.
- Do not do more than you can possibly handle.

✓ Find a balance between giving and taking.

✓ It is okay to say no.
- It makes much more sense to encourage others to help themselves.
- Say no politely but firmly and explain why clearly and convincingly.

✓ Reset interpersonal expectations.

✓ Do not overreach.

✓ Put all of this into action – from now on.

EFFECTIVE DELEGATION

▶ Effective delegation frees up time: It increases effectiveness, eases pressure and reduces stress.

TIPS FOR EFFECTIVE DELEGATION

✓ In the short run, delegation is a pain: You will have to instruct others.

✓ In the long run, delegation is a gain: Others will have to help you.
- You have much less time pressure.
- Others have much more job satisfaction.
- The organisation has an increased performance.

✓ Delegate the entire task to a single person as this increases clarity, motivation and ownership.

✓ Delegation involves not only granting authority but also providing the knowledge, skills and tools to be confident, successful and effective.

✓ You must ensure that the delegate is both qualified and capable of carrying out a particular duty because patient safety has top priority.

✓ Delegate to employees whose competence and judgement you trust.

✓ Give clarity, autonomy, authority and support to the delegate.
✓ Expect commitment, performance, results and responsibility from the delegate.

✓ Avoid misunderstandings and ambiguities by obtaining a clear agreement, in writing, about the delegated assignment.

✓ Instil confidence by offering to be there as a sounding board and safety net.

✓ Monitor the delegated tasks closely.
✓ Provide feedback to the delegate.

✓ Do not interrupt, interfere or intervene unless you really have to.

✓ Do not take back the task, because this could leave the delegate dejected, confused or insulted.

✓ You cannot delegate your accountability.
  • You are still responsible for the success or failure of the task.
  • You must stay in control, on top of things and in charge.

EFFECTIVE READING

▶ Basic criteria for effective selection
- Author
- Argument
- Evidence
- Quality

TIPS FOR EFFECTIVE READING

✓ Encourage your team to present reports and reviews clearly and concisely.

✓ Ask for short summaries, and send succinct replies.

✓ Take yourself off the circulation list for useless information.

✓ Ask yourself: Do I really need to read it? If yes, read blurb, contents, headings and summaries.

✓ Then ask yourself: Do I really need to read more? If yes, read only the important chapters, recommendations and action points.

✓ Read diagonally: Skim the text and pick the cherries. Focus on the beginning and end of each section and on the beginning and end of each paragraph.

EFFECTIVE WRITING

▶ ABC rule for business writing
- A: Effective business writing is accurate.
- B: Effective business writing is brief.
- C: Effective business writing is clear.

▶ Short checklist for business writing
- Purpose of document
- Recipient of document
- Order of contents
- Completeness of contents
- Clarity of language
- Correctness of language

▶ Assertive statements for business writing
- 'I' messages
- To the point
- Brief
- Firm
- Supported with facts
- Positive undertone

▶ Conclusions and recommendations must be based on facts and evidence.

▶ Effective business writing is characterised by crystal clear messages.

TIPS FOR EFFECTIVE WRITING

✓ Compiling possibilities: Use brainstorming.
- Brainstorming results in topic lists.

✓ Giving structure: Use clustering.
- Clustering results in concept maps.

✓ Developing frameworks: Use outlining.
- Outlining results in detailed plans.

✓ Keep it structured and logical.
✓ Keep it direct and powerful.
✓ Keep it short and simple.

✓ Use plain language.
✓ Use common words.
✓ Use clear headings.
✓ Use clear paragraphs.
✓ Use short sentences.
✓ Use short transitions.
✓ Use active voice.
✓ Use personal pronouns.

✓ Avoid abbreviations.
✓ Avoid clichés.
✓ Avoid gobbledegook.

✓ No repetition.
✓ No unnecessary details.
✓ No padding.

✓ Make sure that your language is not aggressive, evasive, stiff, too effusive, too cautious or too defensive.

✓ Present your text in an understandable, professional and accessible way.
✓ Present your text using an attractive, consistent and modern layout.

✓ Check for grammar.
✓ Check for spelling.
✓ Check for capitalisation.
✓ Check for punctuation.

✓ Use a dictionary.
✓ Use a thesaurus.

✓ Revise and edit.

✓ Email
- Do you really need to draft a new email?
- Do you really need to respond to an email?

....

✓ Email
- Keep it concise and precise.
- Use the subject line to deliver the essentials of your message.
- Keep it specific and unambiguous.

....

✓ Email
- Check the salutation for correctness.
- Check the attachments for correctness.

LIFE GOALS

▶ Life is what we make it – always has been, always will be. Of that there is no doubt.

TIPS FOR LIFE GOALS

✓ Always remember your life goals.
- What matters to you in life?
- What are your deepest values and strategic objectives in priority order?
- What do you want to achieve?

....

✓ Develop your dream.

....

✓ Have a laugh.

....

✓ Spread happiness.

....

✓ Enjoy life.

43 HEALTHCARE PERFORMANCE

CHAPTER OVERVIEW

▶ RESPONSIBILITIES
- PROFESSIONAL SUPERVISION
- CLINICAL SUPERVISION
- MANAGERIAL SUPERVISION
- LINE MANAGER AND PERFORMANCE MANAGEMENT

▶ MANAGEMENT
- PERFORMANCE MANAGEMENT RATIONALE
- PERFORMANCE MANAGEMENT SYSTEM
- PERFORMANCE MANAGEMENT CYCLE
- PERFORMANCE MANAGEMENT SCOPE
- PERFORMANCE MANAGEMENT PROCESS
- PERFORMANCE MANAGEMENT IMPACT

▶ IMPLEMENTATION
- PERFORMANCE MANAGEMENT
- SUPPORTING PROCESSES
- SUCCESS FACTORS
- SUCCESS INDICATORS
- JUDGING CRITERIA
- MANAGEMENT TECHNIQUES
- SETTING GOALS
- CONTINUOUS FEEDBACK
- REGULAR APPRAISAL
- REWARDING ACHIEVEMENT

▶ IMPROVEMENT
- TIPS FOR PERFORMANCE IMPROVEMENT

▶ APPRAISAL
- DEFINITION

- IMPACT
- PURPOSE
- METHOD
- PRINCIPLES
- FRAMEWORK
- GUIDELINES
- ASPECTS
- CONVERSATION
- RECORDS
- CONSEQUENCES
- TIPS FOR APPRAISALS

▶ CHALLENGES
- MANAGEMENT OF DIFFICULT EMPLOYEES
- INDICATORS OF NEGATIVISM
- MANAGEMENT OF NEGATIVISM
- TYPES OF BULLYING
- IMPACT OF BULLYING
- MANAGEMENT OF BULLYING
- MANAGEMENT OF UNJUSTIFIED AND EXCESSIVE COMPLAINING AND WHINING
- MANAGEMENT OF PROCRASTINATION
- MANAGEMENT OF MANIPULATION
- MANAGEMENT OF DIFFICULT CONDITIONS
- MANAGEMENT OF CONFLICT
- TIPS FOR EFFECTIVE CONFLICT MANAGEMENT
- MANAGEMENT OF GROUPTHINK
- MANAGEMENT OF ABSENCE
- MANAGEMENT OF TURNOVER

▶ UNDERPERFORMANCE
- INDICATORS OF CHANGE IN PERFORMANCE
- MANAGEMENT OF CHANGE IN PERFORMANCE
- INDICATORS OF UNDERPERFORMANCE
- EVIDENCE FOR UNDERPERFORMANCE
- REASONS FOR UNDERPERFORMANCE
- MANAGEMENT OF UNDERPERFORMANCE
- CONVERSATION ABOUT UNDERPERFORMANCE

- PERFORMANCE IMPROVEMENT PLAN
- MENTORING
- COACHING
- MANAGEMENT OF UNDERPERFORMANCE DUE TO DISABILITY
- MANAGEMENT OF UNDERPERFORMANCE DUE TO HEALTH
- MANAGEMENT OF UNDERPERFORMANCE DUE TO DISPUTES

▶ EXCELLENCE
- INDICATORS OF EXCELLENCE
- MANAGEMENT OF EXCELLENCE
- CONVERSATION ABOUT EXCELLENCE
- TIPS FOR MANAGING EXCELLENCE

43.1. RESPONSIBILITIES

PROFESSIONAL SUPERVISION

▶ Supporting, assuring and developing the knowledge, skills and values of an individual, a team or a service

▶ Benefits of professional supervision for staff, service users and providers

▶ Clinical supervision
▶ Managerial supervision

CLINICAL SUPERVISION

▶ Aims of clinical supervision
- Discussing individual cases
- Reflecting on practice
- Identifying developmental needs
- Reviewing professional standards
- Meeting professional requirements
- Improving service quality

▶ Principles of clinical supervision
- Safety
- Trust
- Confidentiality
  - Exception: Concerns about conduct, competence or health of a supervisee

▶ Benefits of clinical supervision
- Job satisfaction
- Reduced turnover
- Improved retention
- Staff effectiveness
- Improved quality
- Increased accountability
- Patient safety

MANAGERIAL SUPERVISION

▶ Aims of managerial supervision
- Setting objectives
- Setting priorities
- Identifying developmental needs
- Monitoring performance
- Appraising performance

LINE MANAGER AND PERFORMANCE MANAGEMENT

▶ The line manager is responsible for performance management.

▶ The line manager is responsible for managing and leading his/her employees, from the moment they join his/her team.

▶ Roles and responsibilities of the line manager need to be clearly defined, agreed, communicated and implemented.

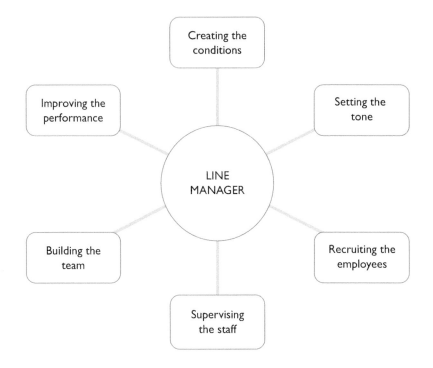

43.2. MANAGEMENT

PERFORMANCE MANAGEMENT RATIONALE

▶ Performance requires more than most employees are willing to do, but no more than they are capable of doing.

▶ Performance management is a continuous process to ensure that employees
  • Realise their full potential
  • Are working to the best of their ability
  • Promote the workplace values

▶ Managers are in the key position to influence employees' performance.

▶ Performance management is an ongoing honest and open two-way communication between manager and employee.

PERFORMANCE MANAGEMENT SYSTEM

▶ Job description
▶ Comprehensive induction
▶ Effective supervision
▶ Professional development
▶ Regular appraisal

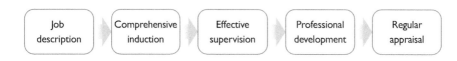

▶ Measurement of performance by means of indicators
  • SMART targets and criteria

PERFORMANCE MANAGEMENT CYCLE

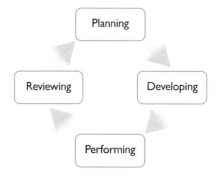

PERFORMANCE MANAGEMENT SCOPE

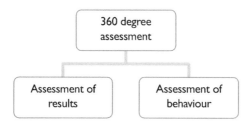

241

PERFORMANCE MANAGEMENT PROCESS

▶ Meaningful engagement with employees
▶ Regular conversations with employees
▶ Clear expectations of desired performance
▶ Constructive feedback on actual performance
▶ Adequate support for employees
▶ Role modelling for employees

PERFORMANCE MANAGEMENT IMPACT

▶ Learning
▶ Development
▶ Quality
▶ Outcome
▶ Governance
▶ Safeguarding

▶ Staff engagement
▶ Staff costs
▶ Patient care
▶ Patient satisfaction
▶ CQC ratings
▶ Financial ratings

▶ Productivity
▶ Profitability

▶ It is important to note, however, that patients and staff want leadership and management to believe in something beyond maximising productivity and optimising profitability.

43.3. IMPLEMENTATION

PERFORMANCE MANAGEMENT

▶ Familiarising oneself with the systems, specific policies and procedures of the organisation
- Human resources
- Supervision meetings
- Performance appraisals

▶ Developing oneself into a leader, role model and mentor of the service
- Visibility
- Approachability
- Supervision
- Informal reviews
- Continuous feedback
- Change management

▶ Getting it right from the start

▶ Improving future performance rather than punishing past performance

▶ Embarking on a continuous journey of performance management

SUPPORTING PROCESSES

▶ Induction

▶ Advice

▶ Guidance

▶ Training

▶ Regulations

▶ Policies

▶ Procedures

▶ Supervision

▶ Feedback

▶ Appraisal

SUCCESS FACTORS

▶ Organisation
- Workplace culture
- Team culture
- Management by example
- Leadership by example

▶ Employees
- Understanding the purpose of their role
- Working towards achieving their objectives
- Taking clear responsibility for their performance

▶ Motivators
- Accountability
- Achievement
- Affiliation
- Communication
- Conditions
- Pay
- Pride
- Promotion
- Recognition
- Relationships
- Remit
- Responsibility

▶ Employees work hard for their salary, even harder for a person, but hardest for a vision.
- A vision is a purpose, an overarching goal, a perspective.

SUCCESS INDICATORS

▶ Staff happiness
- Motivation level
- Stress level

► Staff wellbeing
- Attendance level
- Lateness level
- Absence level

► Staff loyalty
- Exit level
- Turnover level

► Staff engagement levels
- Level 1: Excluded
- Level 2: Expectant
- Level 3: Energised
- Level 4: Expanded
- Level 5: Embedded

► High performing staff
- Committed
- Empowered
- Encouraged
- Engaged
- Enthusiastic
- Equipped
- Inspired
- Involved
- Motivated
- Supported
- Valued

JUDGING CRITERIA

► Functional skills
- Using information
- Communicating effectively

▶ Employability skills
- Solving problems
- Managing oneself
- Working with others
- Acting with responsibility

▶ Goals
▶ Objectives
▶ Requirements
▶ Expectations
▶ Values
▶ Behaviours

MANAGEMENT TECHNIQUES

| Setting goals | Continuous feedback | Regular appraisal | Rewarding achievement |

SETTING GOALS

▶ Selection of goals
- Priority A: High value and major importance
- Priority B: Medium value and secondary importance
- Priority C: Low value and minor importance

▶ Criteria of goals
- SMART goals and objectives
  - Specific
  - Measurable
  - Achievable
  - Relevant
  - Timed

▶ Criteria of goals
- Reasonable
- Challenging
- Demanding
- Reachable
- Fair

▶ Approaches to goals
- Top-down approach to goal setting
- Bottom-up approach to goal setting
- Various combinations of both approaches

▶ Achievement of goals
- Each goal should be broken down into specific tasks, defined outcomes, a timetable and a plan.

▶ Measurement of achievement
- Use of clear performance metrics
  - Performance metrics allow objective assessment of goal achievement.

CONTINUOUS FEEDBACK

▶ Purpose
- Reinforcing good practice
- Clarifying performance expectations
- Highlighting improvement needs

▶ Attributes
- Constructive
- Motivating
- Timely
- Fact based
- Straightforward
- Explicit
- Clear

REGULAR APPRAISAL

▶ Formal performance review/formal performance assessment
- Goals and objectives
- Performance and development
- Self-assessment
- Career aspirations
- Work plan

REWARDING ACHIEVEMENT

▶ Types of rewards
- Financial
- Non-financial
  - Achievement
  - Mastery
  - Recognition
  - Influence
  - Responsibility
  - Autonomy
  - Trust

▶ Communication of rewards
- Hospital intranet
- Social media
  - Facebook
  - Instagram
  - LinkedIn
  - Snapchat
  - Twitter
  - Viber
  - WhatsApp
  - YouTube
- Internal events
- Benefit champions

43.4. IMPROVEMENT

TIPS FOR PERFORMANCE IMPROVEMENT

✓ Lead and manage your employees in a way that gets the best out of them.

✓ Make time for performance improvement.

✓ Create a mindset of high ambition for the employee, the team and the organisation.

✓ Encourage your employees to want more, to think more, to learn more, to know more, to do more and to achieve more, because people always rise to a challenge.

✓ Involve your employees.
✓ Raise the game.
✓ Stretch your employees.
  • Keep your employees stretched, but not stressed.

✓ Remove any barriers to performance, wherever possible.

✓ Think about your employees not only as employees but as people.
✓ A culture characterised by 'kiss up, kick down' is extremely toxic.
✓ Be polite to all employees.
✓ Treat all employees as special.

✓ Make sure your employees know exactly what is expected of them.

✓ Agree clear performance goals.
✓ Agree really realistic targets.
✓ Agree precise quality indicators.
✓ Agree clear performance metrics.

✓ Let employees know exactly where they stand.

....

✓ Note that there is a difference between activities and results.
  • Value results, not activities.
  • Reward outcomes, not promises.

....

✓ Beware of overrating employees.

....

✓ Praise high performance.
✓ Challenge mediocrity.
✓ Address low performance.

....

✓ Attack a problem – not a person.
✓ Address criticism to the wrongdoing – not to the individual.
✓ Relate to facts – not to emotions.

....

✓ Your corrective feedback should be specific, concrete, timely, precise, meaningful and actionable – and it should be given in private, not in public.

....

✓ It is not only what you say but also the way you say it.

....

✓ Do clearly communicate positive feelings.
✓ Do not overcommunicate negative feelings.

....

✓ Use the sandwich approach: Begin and end the feedback talk on a positive note.

....

✓ Do not use hyperbolic language.
✓ Do not make inflammatory statements.

....

✓ Do not make a mountain out of a molehill.

✓ Always act with sound judgement.

✓ Do not take a sledgehammer to crack a nut.

....

✓ Stick to issues that really matter for the organisation.

....

✓ Manage unsettling emotions so that the employees can focus their energy on delivering great care.

....

✓ Acting too emotionally will leave you looking and feeling like an amateur.

....

✓ Listen attentively.

✓ Communicate without interrupting.

✓ Talk it through.

✓ Think it over.

✓ Pause before replying.

✓ Decide consistently.

....

✓ Always ask and listen before answering and deciding, because asking and listening might change your perception of the performance.

....

✓ Be honest.

✓ Be straight.

✓ Be supportive.

✓ Be positive.

....

✓ Avoid negative communication: Challenges, obstacles, barriers …

✓ Use positive communication: Goals, vision, results …

....

✓ Encourage a problem-solving attitude.

✓ Orient feedback towards results.

✓ Praise a results-oriented behaviour.

....

✓ Be objective.

✓ Be fair.

✓ Be consistent.

- Decision fairness – being consistent with different employees on similar issues – improves job commitment, job satisfaction and job performance.

✓ Be impartial.

✓ Be unbiased.

....

✓ Be sensitive and constructive.

✓ Be explicit and specific.

- Do not give mixed signals.

✓ Be supportive and encouraging.

....

✓ Deliver equality.

✓ Do not discriminate against employees.

✓ Value diversity.

....

✓ Manage with fairness.

✓ Do not take sides. Decide on the basis of fact and evidence.

✓ Take positive action.

- Focus on required improvement.
- Focus on desired outcome.
- Focus on constructive advice.

....

✓ Be confident.

✓ Handle stress well.

✓ Be resilient.

....

✓ Ultimately people do what they want to do.

✓ Accept that you cannot change another person's personality and character, despite your best intentions and support.

✓ Protect yourself and do not take it personally.

....

✓ Practise some kind of emotional detachment so that other people's behaviour does not bother you too much.

....

✓ Do not be a myopic leader.
  - See the bigger picture.
  - See the broader perspective.
  - See the better future.
✓ Do not be a micromanaging leader.
  - Live for your mission.
  - Live for your vision.
  - Live for your strategy.

43.5. APPRAISAL

DEFINITION

▶ Framework for measuring actual job performance against specific job objectives

IMPACT

▶ Important part of the overall success of a health organisation

PURPOSE

▶ Monitoring the progress and achievement of the organisation
▶ Supporting the performance and development of the organisation

▶ Valuing employees
▶ Encouraging employees
▶ Motivating employees
▶ Supporting employees

▶ Recognising what the employee has achieved
▶ Identifying how the employee can develop

METHOD

▶ Formal conversation with every staff member at regular intervals

▶ Two-way process between appraiser and appraisee

PRINCIPLES

▶ Appraisal should be a continuous process, not a compulsory exercise.

▶ Appraiser and appraisee
- Good relationship
- Mutual trust
- Positive intention

▶ Establishing trust
▶ Setting the right tone
▶ Listening with full attention
▶ Encouraging the appraisee
▶ Reaching a genuine agreement
▶ Discussing the next steps
▶ Maintaining confidentiality

FRAMEWORK

▶ Job description
▶ Person specification

GUIDELINES

▶ Key guidelines for managing doctors
- General Medical Council
- Revalidation and appraisal
  - Licensed doctors to be up to date and fit to practise

ASPECTS

▶ Organisational goals
▶ Departmental goals
▶ Individual goals

▶ Achievement
▶ Progress
▶ Potential

CONVERSATION

▶ Basic principles
- Setting a time
- Preparing the records
- Gathering information
- Collecting evidence
- Clarifying the aims
- Conducting the conversation
  - Agreeing an overall agenda
  - Reviewing the previous appraisal
  - Referring to targets
  - Discussing general progress
  - Recognising achievements
  - Identifying organisational issues
  - Agreeing new objectives
  - Agreeing an action plan
  - Recording all agreed outcomes

▶ Detailed topics
- Past performance
  - Review of performance and development against goals and objectives
  - Review of the tasks section of the job description
  - Review of knowledge and skills requirements of job description and related person specification
  - Review of learning and training to support the achievement of goals and objectives

- Future requirements
  - New goals and objectives
  - Areas for knowledge and skills development linked to job requirements and business needs
  - Career and personal aspirations

RECORDS

▶ Key achievements
  - Collected evidence
▶ Targets met
▶ Areas for improvement
  - Person related
  - Job related
  - Organisation related
▶ New targets
▶ Action plan
  - Manageable phases

▶ Managers should keep a record of the performance achievements, successes and challenges of their employees.
  - The manager should share the record with the employee.

CONSEQUENCES

▶ Performance shortfalls should be addressed immediately.
▶ Performance changes should be managed effectively.
▶ Consistently good performance should be highlighted and acknowledged.
▶ Exceptionally good performance should be nurtured and rewarded.

TIPS FOR APPRAISALS

✓ Explain the intention of the appraisal to the employee.

✓ Ensure the appraisal is seen as purposeful, meaningful, constructive and productive.

✓ Discuss achievements, challenges and aspirations.

✓ Convey a sense of purpose to stimulate discretionary efforts from employees.

✓ Inspire your employees to take responsibility for their own development and continuous improvement.

✓ Encourage self-awareness, willingness to learn, flexibility to act and self-initiative.

✓ Do not impose your own views.
✓ Do not dictate your own ideas.
✓ Do not implement your own solutions.

✓ Empower the employee.
✓ Negotiate the goals.
✓ Agree the objectives.

✓ Do not say: 'You have done everything right. Keep going.'
✓ Do not say: 'You are not good enough. Do better.'
✓ Do say: 'You have come this far. Where are you going now?'
✓ Do say: 'You should do … by … in this way … to progress further.'

✓ Finally, the best question to ask yourself as an appraiser is: How would you like to be appraised?

43.6. CHALLENGES

MANAGEMENT OF DIFFICULT EMPLOYEES

▶ Difficult behaviours, attitudes, personalities and characters
- Negativism
- Bullying
- Unjustified and excessive complaining and whining
- Procrastination
- Manipulation

INDICATORS OF NEGATIVISM

▶ 'No' attitude
▶ 'I cannot' attitude
▶ 'Not now' attitude
▶ 'But' attitude
- Declining to do something
- Doing the opposite of something
- Doing something utterly at variance
- Preventing something being done

▶ Being pessimistic
▶ Emphasising their problems
▶ Avoiding constructive discussion
▶ Acting selfishly
▶ Looking for the bad
▶ Belittling other employees' accomplishments
▶ Focusing only on criticism
▶ Pulling down other people
▶ Shying away
▶ Refusing team activities
▶ Criticising their superiors
▶ Being secretive

MANAGEMENT OF NEGATIVISM

▶ Investing some time
▶ Being courteous
▶ Listening intently
▶ Involving the employee
▶ Understanding the issues
▶ Addressing the concerns
▶ Asking for solutions
▶ Providing help
▶ Acting assertively
▶ Taking a decision

▶ Stopping disruptive behaviour by introducing consequences

TYPES OF BULLYING

▶ Undermining behaviour
▶ Persistent criticism
▶ Threats
▶ Aggression

IMPACT OF BULLYING

▶ Low care quality
▶ Low organisational effectiveness
▶ Damage to reputation
▶ Costs of litigation
▶ High absence levels
▶ High staff turnover

MANAGEMENT OF BULLYING

▶ Awareness of workplace bullying
▶ Training the entire workforce
  • Systematic staff empowerment

- Raising concerns
- Zero tolerance for even small acts of unprofessional behaviour
  - Anything less than professional is absolutely unacceptable.
    - Taking immediate action
    - Challenging rude behaviour
    - Following regulations, policies and procedures
    - Promoting equality, diversity and inclusion
    - Preventing further harm
    - Taking disciplinary action
- Intervening speedily
- Improving the organisational climate
  - Positive workplace culture
- Focusing on preventive action

MANAGEMENT OF UNJUSTIFIED AND EXCESSIVE COMPLAINING AND WHINING

- Staying away
- Not reacting
- Setting high standards for good manners
- Using appropriate motivational signs
- Modelling the opposite behaviour
- Asking the complainer for a solution
- Not commenting
- Moving on

MANAGEMENT OF PROCRASTINATION

- Analysing the causes of procrastination
- Providing training in time management
- Adapting a results oriented leadership style
- Asking for frequent updates on progress
- Specific coaching
- Setting deadlines

MANAGEMENT OF MANIPULATION

▶ Disclosing manipulation
▶ Analysing the impact on the organisation
▶ Preventing harm
▶ Making records and taking disciplinary action

MANAGEMENT OF DIFFICULT CONDITIONS

▶ Difficult conditions
  ● Conflict
  ● Groupthink
  ● Absence
  ● Turnover

MANAGEMENT OF CONFLICT

▶ Types of conflict
  ● Classification I
    ▪ Intrapersonal
    ▪ Interpersonal
    ▪ Intergroup
  ● Classification II
    ▪ Latent
    ▪ Perceived
    ▪ Felt
    ▪ Manifest
    ▪ Suppressed
    ▪ Resolved
  ● Classification III
    ▪ Task based
    ▪ Relationship based
    ▪ Context based

▶ Sources of conflict
- Interpersonal relations
- Conflicting roles
- Ambiguous responsibilities
- Poor communication
- Inadequate information
- Hidden agendas
- Excessive competition
- Unfair treatment
- Limited resources
- Organisational change

▶ Principles
- Climate of informal and early conflict resolution
- Mediation schemes
- Procedures for formal and critical conflict management

▶ Strategies
- Denying
- Avoiding
- Negotiating
- Compromising
- Confronting
- Compelling

▶ Techniques
- Acknowledging the conflict
- Listening attentively
- Accepting feelings
- Communicating empathetically
- Exploring options
- Acting professionally
- Summarising the outcome

▶ Outcomes
- Getting agreement
- Building consensus
- Finding compromises
- Negotiating halfway
- Setting direction

▶ Resolution
- Increased productivity
- Increased morale
- More effective use of time
- More effective use of resources
- Better performance
- Better results

TIPS FOR EFFECTIVE CONFLICT MANAGEMENT

✓ Anticipate conflicts as far as possible. Uncover the reasons behind the conflict.

✓ Prioritise every conflict.
- A – Low importance to you and low importance to the other: Forget it.
- B – Low importance to you and high importance to the other: Give in.
- C – High importance to you and low importance to the other: Strategise. Advocate.
- D – High importance to you and high importance to the other: Cooperate. Compromise.

✓ Tackle issues quickly.

✓ Analyse possible causes.

✓ Approach every conflict with a clear head.

✓ Find joint solutions.

✓ Always remain friendly.

✓ Separate people from conflicts.

✓ Concentrate on people's interests rather than their positions.

✓ Set the right tone.
✓ Adopt a measured approach.
✓ Aim for balanced solutions.

✓ Agree on the small things first – the big things will then follow.

✓ If you cannot reach an agreement, define the way forward. Remember that you are in charge.

MANAGEMENT OF GROUPTHINK

▶ Groupthink implies a lack of diversification in experience, behaviour and outlook.
  • Groupthink gradually leads to a deterioration of mental efficiency and realistic assessment and has disadvantages for the organisation.
    ▪ Self-insulation from contrary perspectives
    ▪ Self-justification of own conclusions
    ▪ Sense of moral superiority
    ▪ Irrationality in decision making
▶ Teams with diverse demographics are invariably a proven remedy for groupthink.

MANAGEMENT OF ABSENCE

▶ Causes
  • Health issues
  • Job design
  • Work attitude
  • Work pattern
  • Employment relations
  • Family responsibilities

▶ Management
- Having absence policies
- Monitoring individual absence
- Seeking medical opinions
- Taking disciplinary action

▶ Employment rights
- Employment law
- Contractual terms
- Organisational policies

▶ Return to work interview

▶ Fit for work referral

▶ Capability procedure

MANAGEMENT OF TURNOVER

▶ Positive impact of employee turnover
- New opportunities
- Fresh thoughts
- Positive changes

▶ Negative impact of employee turnover
- Direct costs
  - Recruitment costs
  - Interviewing costs
  - Training costs
- Indirect costs
  - Workload effects
  - Morale effects
  - Performance effects
- Opportunity costs
  - Knowledge loss
  - Skills loss
  - Abilities loss

43.7. UNDERPERFORMANCE

INDICATORS OF CHANGE IN PERFORMANCE

- ▶ Less interest
- ▶ Less willingness
- ▶ Less engagement
- ▶ Less effort
- ▶ More errors
- ▶ Poor timekeeping
- ▶ Missing deadlines
- ▶ Increased absence

MANAGEMENT OF CHANGE IN PERFORMANCE

- ▶ Fair management
- ▶ Professional management
- ▶ Decisions on the basis of facts and evidence
- ▶ Early action
- ▶ Reasonable action

INDICATORS OF UNDERPERFORMANCE

- ▶ 'Clock watching' attitude
- ▶ 'Just enough' attitude
- ▶ Mental absence
- ▶ Inner resignation

EVIDENCE FOR UNDERPERFORMANCE

- ▶ Performance indicators
- ▶ Concrete incidents
- ▶ Specific examples

REASONS FOR UNDERPERFORMANCE

▶ Lack of capability
  • 'I want to, but I can't.'
▶ Lack of conduct
  • 'I can, but I won't.'

▶ Work related
▶ Non-work related

MANAGEMENT OF UNDERPERFORMANCE

▶ Analysing the root causes of the gaps between actual and expected performance

▶ Focusing on the future, not the past
▶ Focusing on evidence, not on impressions
▶ Focusing on the abilities, not the person
▶ Focusing on continuity, not on appraisals
▶ Focusing on the development, not the performance

▶ Informal approach
  • Day-to-day management
  • One-to-one meetings
▶ Formal approach
  • Disciplinary procedures
    ▪ Performance improvement meeting
    ▪ Formal disciplinary hearing

▶ Serious incidents must be managed using formal procedures because they entail risks to patients, other employees or the organisation.

CONVERSATION ABOUT UNDERPERFORMANCE

▶ Supportive but firm approach

▶ Describing the facts
▶ Finding the causes
▶ Explaining the consequences
▶ Encouraging self-reflection
▶ Agreeing a plan
▶ Re-evaluating the goals
▶ Concluding the discussion

▶ Job-related
▶ Goal-oriented
▶ Non-judgemental
▶ Descriptive
▶ Specific
▶ Detailed

▶ 'I noticed …'
▶ 'This caused …'
▶ 'I have a few concerns …'
▶ 'I have a sensitive issue …'
▶ 'Can you give me your perspective …'
▶ 'Can we agree the following actions …'
▶ 'The outcome of our discussion is …'
▶ 'The consequences of repeated behaviour are …'

▶ Comments should be based on observations, not on assumptions.
▶ They should be underpinned with specific examples, not with vague platitudes.
▶ Feedback should be given without delay, not after ages.

▶ The conversation should always focus on behaviours and attitudes, not on personality and character.

▶ Dignity and respect are key, for both sides.

▶ Conversations about performance (manager's issues/concerns, employee's responses/reactions) should be documented.
   ● Copies of the records should be shared.

PERFORMANCE IMPROVEMENT PLAN

▶ Key questions
   ● What needs to improve?
      ▪ Performance problem
   ● By when?
      ▪ Time frame
   ● Has it actually improved?
      ▪ Progress review

▶ SMART goals and objectives
   ● Specific
   ● Measurable
   ● Achievable
   ● Relevant
   ● Timed

▶ Support
   ● Learning
   ● Training
   ● Mentoring
   ● Coaching
   ● Counselling
   ● Shadowing
▶ Reasonable adjustments
▶ Monitoring

MENTORING

▶ Relationship oriented
▶ Long term
▶ Development driven
▶ No agenda
▶ Broad view
▶ Informal process

COACHING

▶ Task oriented
▶ Short term
▶ Performance driven
▶ Specific agenda
▶ Focused view
▶ Formal process

MANAGEMENT OF UNDERPERFORMANCE DUE TO DISABILITY

▶ Open conversation
▶ Specialist advice
▶ Reasonable adjustments
  • ACAS guidance
▶ Occupational health
▶ Government grant
  • Access to Work
    ▪ Grant for people with a disability, a health condition or a mental health condition

MANAGEMENT OF UNDERPERFORMANCE DUE TO HEALTH

▶ Absence analysis
  • Patterns in the days
  • Themes in the reasons
  • Fit notes
  • Medical reports

- Open conversation
- Return to work interviews
- Occupational health
- Government grant
  - Access to Work
    - Grant for people with a disability, a health condition or a mental health condition

MANAGEMENT OF UNDERPERFORMANCE DUE TO DISPUTES

- Analysis
  - Difference in values?
  - Conflict of interests?
  - Clash of egos?
  - Lack of communication?
- Conversation
  - Participatory methods
  - Passionate stance
  - Respectful approach
  - Fair decisions

43.8. EXCELLENCE

INDICATORS OF EXCELLENCE

- Performing outstandingly
- Always going the extra mile
- Giving discretionary effort
- Taking pride in the job
- Showing loyalty

MANAGEMENT OF EXCELLENCE

- Rewards on the basis of merit
  - Recognition plans
  - Financial rewards

- Health and wellbeing opportunities
- Terms and conditions benefits
- Career progression
- Award schemes

CONVERSATION ABOUT EXCELLENCE

▶ Acknowledging achievements
▶ Showing appreciation
▶ Congratulating
▶ Praising
▶ Encouraging
▶ Discussing aspirations
▶ Giving support

▶ 'I noticed that you …'
▶ 'It really helped us …'
▶ 'Thank you very much …'
▶ 'It is really appreciated …'

TIPS FOR MANAGING EXCELLENCE

✓ Encourage, nurture and value high aspirations, talent and excellent performance.

✓ Invest in top talents relationally.
✓ Treat top talents as your partners.
✓ Move top talents into your inner circle.
✓ Pick top talents for your succession.
✓ Invest in top talents financially.

✓ Align recognition schemes with the organisational objectives.

✓ Apply recognition schemes which have a transparent concept, are within the control of the employee and have a known outcome.

- Demonstrate your commitment and investment in your staff.
- Communicate your reward offer.
- Evaluate your reward package.
- Maximise the impact of rewards for your organisation.

....

✓ Cherish talents: Grant informal surprise bonuses.

....

✓ Create structures for succession to key roles.

44 HEALTHCARE PRODUCTIVITY

CHAPTER OVERVIEW

- ▶ LEVERS OF PRODUCTIVITY
- ▶ WELL ORGANISED WORK
- ▶ TALENT MANAGEMENT
- ▶ SKILLED MANAGERS
- ▶ INFORMED EMPLOYEES
- ▶ CLEARLY DEFINED RIGHTS AND RESPONSIBILITIES
- ▶ HIGH TRUST
- ▶ FAIR TREATMENT
- ▶ HEALTHCARE IT
- ▶ EFFECTIVE CONFLICT MANAGEMENT
- ▶ KILLERS OF PRODUCTIVITY
- ▶ PRODUCTIVITY IMPROVEMENT APPROACHES

LEVERS OF PRODUCTIVITY

- ▶ Well organised work
- ▶ Talent management
- ▶ Skilled managers
- ▶ Informed employees
- ▶ Clearly defined rights and responsibilities
- ▶ High trust
- ▶ Fair treatment
- ▶ Healthcare IT
- ▶ Effective conflict management

WELL ORGANISED WORK

▶ Employer
  - Designing the jobs and work
  - Investing in learning and training
▶ Employee
  - Influencing the working conditions
  - Innovating the service provision

TALENT MANAGEMENT

▶ Talent management is about getting the right people in the right positions and doing the right things.
▶ An organisation where employees are encouraged to develop their potential creates the perfect climate for high productivity.

SKILLED MANAGERS

▶ High concern for productivity combined with high concern for people is most effective.
  - Competent
  - Efficient
  - Confident

INFORMED EMPLOYEES

▶ Employees involved in consultation, decision making and change

CLEARLY DEFINED RIGHTS AND RESPONSIBILITIES

▶ Precise and written statements of rights and responsibilities for employers and employees
  - Clear expectations and values
  - Open and honest communication

HIGH TRUST

▶ Culture of open, transparent and honest communication, information and consultation

FAIR TREATMENT

▶ Employer
- Championing equality
- Valuing diversity
- Promoting inclusion
- Challenging discrimination

▶ Employee
- Feeling safe
- Feeling supported
- Feeling empowered
- Feeling valued
  - Equal pay
  - Fair conditions
  - Recognition of discretionary effort
  - Targeted feedback
  - Personal advancement

HEALTHCARE IT

▶ IT is an enabler of progress and productivity in healthcare.

EFFECTIVE CONFLICT MANAGEMENT

▶ Conflicts in the workplace are almost inevitable.
▶ Successful organisational leadership also includes effective conflict management.
- Avoiding and resolving negative conflict which is disruptive and destructive
▶ Most conflicts need to be dealt with.

KILLERS OF PRODUCTIVITY

▶ Commuting
▶ Emails
▶ Gossip
▶ Internet
▶ Social media
▶ Meetings
▶ Noise
▶ Smartphones
▶ Texting

▶ Bullying
▶ Conflict
▶ Cyberbullying
▶ Discrimination
▶ Disputes
▶ Exclusion
▶ Harassment
▶ Humiliation
▶ Intimidation
▶ Marginalisation
▶ Oppression
▶ Retaliation
▶ Ridicule
▶ Stereotyping
▶ Stigmatisation
▶ Victimisation

PRODUCTIVITY IMPROVEMENT APPROACHES

▶ Healthcare system and healthcare organisations
  • Economic performance review
  • Cost improvement programme

- Outcomes based commissioning
- Quality, innovation, productivity and prevention programme (QIPP)
- Healthcare transformation
- Service redesign
- Contract reviews

▶ Hospital and departments
  - Effective admission management
  - Effective management of the diagnostic services
  - Effective management of intensive care capacities
  - Effective management of the operating department
  - Effective discharge management

▶ Accident and Emergency
  - Constraint management
  - Eligibility thresholds
  - Fast track
  - Queuing analysis
  - Lean management

45 HEALTHCARE TALENTS

CHAPTER OVERVIEW

▶ MANAGEMENT
- TALENT MANAGEMENT
- RECRUITING TALENT
- TIPS FOR RECRUITING TALENT
- POSITIONING TALENT
- EQUIPPING TALENT
- DEVELOPING TALENT
- EMPOWERING TALENT
- RETAINING TALENT
- SUCCESSION PLANNING

▶ INDUCTION
- NEW ROLE
- OVERARCHING PRINCIPLES
- PREPARING
- PRIORITISING
- PLANNING
- TEAM
- KEY RELATIONSHIPS
- PROFILE
- FEEDBACK
- REFLECTING
- REVIEWING

279

45.1. MANAGEMENT

TALENT MANAGEMENT

- ▶ Leadership development
  - Recruiting talent
  - Positioning talent
  - Equipping talent
  - Developing talent
  - Empowering talent
  - Retaining talent
- ▶ Succession planning

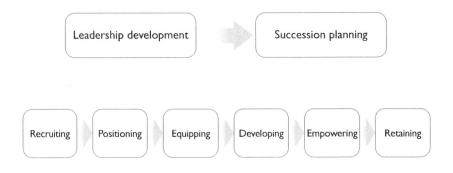

- ▶ The right people, in the right roles, with the right values
  - Creating a productive and sustainable organisation which meets its strategic and operational goals

RECRUITING TALENT

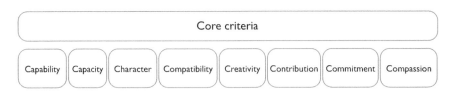

Technical competence		
Knowledge	Experience	Skills

Personal competence		
Aptitude	Attitude	Ability

Interpersonal competence		
Traits	Behaviours	Drivers

▶ Recruiting talent takes time and patience.
▶ A rigorous recruitment process increases the chances of finding great talent.
▶ Great talent is key to success.

▶ Past job performance is the surest indicator of future job performance.

▶ International diversity improves the creativity and productivity of home talent.
  ● Creative processes and productivity gains are driven by different backgrounds, different personalities, different experiences and different viewpoints.

▶ Monochrome recruitment, in contrast, may result in an organisational deadlock.

▶ Diversity among employees makes a team stronger.

▶ Many international applicants are outstandingly courageous, natural risk takers and highly determined.

▶ International vibrancy and entrepreneurial spirit are an asset and a treasure for the whole organisation and the entire workforce.

TIPS FOR RECRUITING TALENT

✓ Recruiting greatness matters.

✓ Attract and value the brightest and the best.

✓ Strive to have several talented candidates to choose from.

✓ Do not recruit only on the basis of knowledge and experience.
✓ Do recruit also on the basis of aptitude and attitude.
✓ You can train the former, but you cannot train the latter.

✓ The absolute importance of due diligence: Do not hire a liar.

✓ Think globally when you recruit.
✓ Make a difference in the fierce competition for talent.
✓ Recruit only high class candidates.

POSITIONING TALENT

▶ A talent can shift and adapt quickly.
▶ A talent manages the different needs and expectations of a diverse workforce.
▶ A talent leads with purpose and meaning.

EQUIPPING TALENT

▶ Investing in employees, enabling them to develop their intellectual flexibility, transferable skills and leadership potential

DEVELOPING TALENT

▶ Aligning talent strategies to the business strategy
▶ Focusing on creative, lateral and strategic thinking
  • Overcoming the constraints of how things have always been done
    ▪ Avoiding fixed thinking
    ▪ Challenging popular thinking
    ▪ Cultivating big picture thinking
    ▪ Harnessing possibility thinking
    ▪ Encouraging disruptive thinking
▶ Offering continuous development to all high potentials

EMPOWERING TALENT

▶ Induction
▶ Training
▶ Support
▶ Encouragement
▶ Respect
▶ Trust

▶ It is all about leveraging creativity.

RETAINING TALENT

▶ Employee value propositions
  • Workplace
  • Career
  • Culture
  • Pay
  • Benefits

▶ Employee value propositions
  • 'Great place'
  • 'Great organisation'

- 'Great job'
- 'Great rewards'
- 'Great fun'

SUCCESSION PLANNING

▶ Ensuring the sustainability of leadership
▶ Developing capability and marketability for a suitable pool of potential candidates
▶ Protecting the organisation from gaps

▶ Developing a leadership pipeline in an organisation

▶ The lasting value of a leader is succession planning.

45.2. INDUCTION

NEW ROLE

Centre stage				
Vision	Workforce	Culture	Governance	Infrastructure

Mixed emotions				
Excitement	Pride	Anticipation	Doubts	Trepidation

▶ The early phase in the new role is the critical period.

▶ The first one hundred days count: They make you or break you. Success or failure. Get it right from the beginning.

▶ Early wins are the greatest boost for your confidence and your reputation.

▶ Performance aspects
  • You are an intellectual being.
  • You are an emotional being.
  • You are a talented being.
  • You are an ambitious being.

▶ Performance acceleration
  • You need to have the better vision.
  • You need to have the better strategy.
  • You need to have the better goals.
  • You need to have the better team.

▶ Insist on being better than you are today.

▶ Overarching principles
▶ Performance framework
  • You need to prepare.
  • You need to prioritise.
  • You need plans.
  • You need a team.
  • You need key relationships.
  • You need a profile.
  • You need feedback.
  • You need to reflect.
  • You need to review.

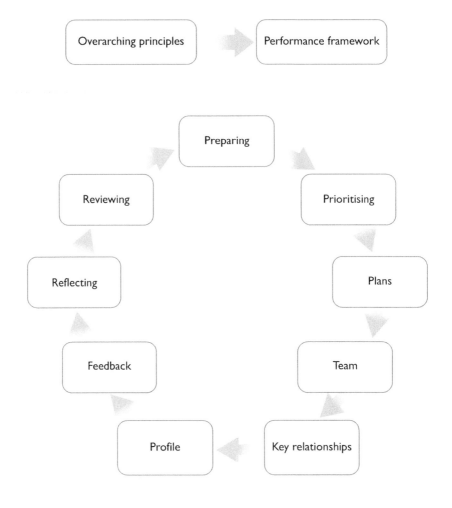

OVERARCHING PRINCIPLES

▶ Keep calm.
▶ Keep confident.
▶ Stay grounded.
▶ Stay centred.

PREPARING

▶ You need all your time, energy and thoughts for the new role.
▶ Therefore, finish with your previous position and concentrate on your new position.
  • Take a break between jobs.

▶ You need all your commitment, dedication and focus for the new job.

▶ Take care of your physical, emotional, mental and spiritual needs.

▶ Allow time to sit back and relax.
▶ Allow time to work out and exercise.

▶ Eat healthily.
▶ Move more.
▶ Sleep better.
▶ Avoid alcohol.
▶ Abstain from smoking.
▶ Improve relationships.
▶ Manage stress.
▶ Worry less.
▶ Succeed better.

▶ Keep fit, exercise regularly and stay trim: *Mens sana in corpore sano.*

▶ Do not burn the candle at both ends.

PRIORITISING

▶ When faced with multiple issues, identify the most important.

▶ Understand the key challenges.
▶ Set the right priorities.
▶ Concentrate on the core issues.
▶ Focus on the desired outcomes.

▶ Do not ignore problems.
▶ Do not sweep anything under the carpet.

► Deal with the issues.

► Focus on your strategy.
  • No chaotic fire-fighting, no doing things for the sake of doing things, no task-driven priorities.
► Concentrate on your goals.

► Start with the end in mind: What do you ultimately want to achieve?

PLANNING

► Which tasks do you need to stop?
► Which tasks do you need to continue?
► Which tasks do you need to start?

► How to be a unique contributor
► How to be a value adder
► How to be a performance achiever
► How to be a transition maker
► How to be a culture changer
► How to be a successful leader

► Which relationship building?
► Which communication architecture?
► Which leadership culture?

TEAM

► Who conceives something?
► Who believes in something?
► Who achieves something?

- ▶ Who is an analyst?
- ▶ Who is a creative?
- ▶ Who is an improver?
- ▶ Who is a facilitator?
- ▶ Who is an administrator?

- ▶ Who has personality?
- ▶ Who has principles?
- ▶ Who has purpose?
- ▶ Who has plans?
- ▶ Who has priorities?
- ▶ Who has passion?
- ▶ Who has power?
- ▶ Who has performance?

- ▶ Who stays?
- ▶ Who else is needed?
- ▶ Who will fit in?
- ▶ Who leaves?

- ▶ Your team is your greatest asset: It is important that your team deeply respects and trusts you.

- ▶ Build rapport.
- ▶ Build commitment.
- ▶ Build credibility.
- ▶ Build respect.
- ▶ Build trust.

- ▶ Know your team and how it works.
- ▶ Align your team and make it strong.

▶ Position the team members properly.
  - Where do they add most value?
  - Where do they have most success?

▶ Give clear guidelines.
▶ Give professional autonomy.
▶ Give freedom and trust.
▶ Give individual control.
▶ Give clear feedback.

▶ On the one hand, let go and trust your team.
▶ On the other hand, hold on and supervise your team.
  - Find the right balance between the two.

▶ Let your team take ownership.

▶ Make your team feel good.

▶ Celebrate accomplishments with your team.

KEY RELATIONSHIPS

▶ It is all about people and their relationships: Who matters? And why?

▶ Invest in a strong network of key influencers, stakeholders, gatekeepers and decision makers.

▶ Networks are personal, strategic or operational.
▶ Networks help individuals to become better connected, better equipped and better known.
▶ Networks take time, patience and effort.

▶ Networks focus on common interests.

▶ Networks need to be maintained
  - Internally and externally
  - With superiors, peers and inferiors
  - Continuously and comprehensively

▶ Do you know the formal and informal networks?
▶ Do you read between the lines?
▶ Do you understand the overt and covert agendas?
▶ Do you check below the surface?

▶ Identify potential competitors.
▶ Identify potential accelerators.
▶ Identify potential blockers.

PROFILE

▶ Start as a leader, not as a manager.

▶ Lead, deliver and succeed immediately: Progress needs speed.

▶ Concentrate on early wins and make a powerful impression.

▶ Take control.
▶ Expect surprises.
▶ Avoid mistakes.
▶ Set direction.
▶ Gain followers.
▶ Communicate effectively.
▶ Deliver results.
▶ Fuel momentum.

- ▶ Shape culture.
- ▶ Sustain progress.

- ▶ Keep track of everything you say, write and do.

- ▶ Maximise opportunity by persevering in doing the right thing.

FEEDBACK

- ▶ Ask for feedback regularly.
- ▶ Check and reconfirm expectations and priorities with board and stakeholders.
- ▶ Review progress against plan.

REFLECTING

- ▶ Lessons learned?
- ▶ Progress recorded?
- ▶ Achievements communicated?
- ▶ Success celebrated?
- ▶ Satisfaction achieved?

REVIEWING

- ▶ Desired outcomes obtained?
- ▶ New aspirations created?
- ▶ Next steps planned?

- ▶ After your first great success, do not rest on your laurels, but follow it up with two more.

- ▶ Success is to know and do something that nobody else knows and does.

46 HEALTHCARE TEAMS

CHAPTER OVERVIEW

- ▶ LEADING A TEAM
- ▶ EFFECTIVE TEAM WORKING
- ▶ EFFECTIVE TEAM SYNERGY
- ▶ EFFECTIVE TEAM RESULTS
- ▶ EFFECTIVE TEAM RELATIONSHIPS
- ▶ TIPS FOR EXECUTIVES

LEADING A TEAM

- ▶ Knowing the team members as people
  - Backgrounds
  - Concerns
  - Desires
  - Dreams
  - Emotions
  - Needs
  - Plans
  - Preferences
  - Views
  - Wishes
- ▶ Treating the team members as individuals

- ▶ Agreeing and sharing common goals
- ▶ Directing and empowering the team members
- ▶ Supporting and assisting the team members

▶ Motivating and inspiring the team members
▶ Encouraging and valuing individual contributions

▶ Thinking about each individual in the team
▶ Being sensitive to individuality
▶ Adapting the leadership style to each individual

▶ Creating conditions for inspiration and growth
▶ Presenting teams with a vision and a strategy
▶ Giving feedback on progress and performance

▶ Promoting human rights
▶ Promoting equality
▶ Promoting diversity
▶ Promoting inclusion
▶ Promoting global thinking

▶ Promoting complementary skills and strengths

▶ Addressing dysfunctional team dynamics

EFFECTIVE TEAM WORKING

▶ Strong leadership
▶ Competent members
▶ Clear identity
▶ Defined roles
▶ Collaborative culture
▶ High trust
▶ Shared objectives
▶ Excellent standards
▶ Unified commitment
▶ Effective communication

EFFECTIVE TEAM SYNERGY

▶ Managing talent
▶ Reaching potential
▶ Establishing norms
▶ Shaping purpose
▶ Developing momentum
▶ Unleashing creativity
▶ Giving inspiration
▶ Taking risks
▶ Balancing shortcomings
▶ Overcoming conflict

EFFECTIVE TEAM RESULTS

▶ Every team member contributes.
▶ Every team member benefits.
▶ The organisation is a winner.
▶ The patient is the champion.

EFFECTIVE TEAM RELATIONSHIPS

▶ Excellent in-team relationships are as important as excellent inter-team relationships – because no team works in isolation.
  • Mutual respect, trust and benefit are paramount.

TIPS FOR EXECUTIVES

✓ Promote team diversity.
✓ Champion divergent thinking.
✓ Emphasise where complementary strengths combine to create high performance.
✓ Highlight team achievements.
✓ Celebrate joint success.

✓ Practise strengths-based delegation.

....

✓ Rotate some responsibilities within the team to show mutual respect.

....

✓ Make your team feel valued.

....

✓ Remember: There is no organisational success without the team's full endorsement.

47 HEALTHCARE MANAGERS

CHAPTER OVERVIEW

- ▶ QUALIFICATION
  - ROLE AND RESPONSIBILITIES
  - CAPABILITIES AND QUALITIES
  - KEY SUCCESS FACTORS
  - REGISTRATION OF MANAGERS
  - RESOURCES FOR MANAGERS
- ▶ STANDARDS
  - GOVERNANCE
    - LEGISLATION, STANDARDS AND FRAMEWORKS
    - GOVERNANCE DEFINITION
    - GOVERNANCE CRITERIA
  - CONDUCT
    - CONDUCT CODE FOR NHS MANAGERS
    - SEVEN PRINCIPLES OF PUBLIC LIFE
    - SIX C'S OF HEALTHCARE EXCELLENCE
- ▶ INDUCTION
  - INDUCTION STANDARDS
  - GOVERNANCE AND ACCOUNTABILITY
  - INFORMATION AND COMMUNICATION
  - RELATIONSHIPS AND PARTNERSHIPS
  - PATIENT CENTRED PRACTICE
  - TEAM ORIENTED MANAGEMENT
  - FINANCES AND RESOURCES
  - EQUALITY AND DIVERSITY
  - SAFEGUARDING AND PROTECTION
  - PROFESSIONAL DEVELOPMENT
  - CHANGE MANAGEMENT

- **BUSINESS MANAGEMENT**
- **QUALITY ASSURANCE**
- **MANAGEMENT PROCESS**
▶ **DEVELOPMENT**
  - **PROFESSIONAL DEVELOPMENT**

47.1. QUALIFICATION

ROLE AND RESPONSIBILITIES

▶ Managers are the lead professionals in the service.
▶ Managers set the standard of the service.
▶ Managers are the role models for the workforce.

CAPABILITIES AND QUALITIES

▶ Managers should be people who are
  - Capable
  - Skilled
  - Confident
▶ Managers should be people who show
  - Imagination
  - Enthusiasm
  - Determination

KEY SUCCESS FACTORS

▶ Managers should constantly reflect on whether they are doing the very best that can be done: the right services, in the right way, at the right time, in the right place and with the right results.

REGISTRATION OF MANAGERS

▶ CQC registers managers of regulated activities.
▶ The registered manager is responsible and accountable for compliance with the relevant regulation.

▶ Essential requirements relating to registered managers
  - Good character
  - Necessary qualifications, skills and experience
  - Proper health
  - Information specified in Schedule 3
    ▪ Proof of identity
    ▪ Evidence of conduct
    ▪ Criminal record certificate
      - Disclosure and Barring Service (DBS) check
    ▪ Full employment history
    ▪ Documentation of qualifications

▶ Managers and CQC
  - Registered managers must be fit and proper persons with the necessary qualifications and experience.

▶ Certification of the Faculty of Medical Leadership and Management
  - Fellowship
  - Senior Fellowship
    ▪ Assessment of knowledge, behaviours, experience and impact

RESOURCES FOR MANAGERS

▶ Relevant organisations
▶ Essential reading
▶ Trusted websites
▶ Professional networks
▶ Line managers
▶ Legal advisers

▶ Academy of Medical Royal Colleges
▶ Advisory, Conciliation and Arbitration Service
▶ Care Quality Commission
▶ Chartered Institute of Personnel and Development
▶ Citizens Advice

▶ Department of Health and Social Care
▶ Equality and Human Rights Commission
▶ Faculty of Medical Leadership and Management
▶ General Medical Council
▶ Good Governance Institute
▶ Health Education England
▶ Health Foundation
▶ Healthcare Financial Management Association
▶ Healthcare Information and Management Systems Society
▶ Healthcare Quality Improvement Partnership
▶ Healthcare Safety Investigation Branch
▶ Investors in People
▶ King's Fund
▶ National Clinical Assessment Service
▶ National Institute for Health and Care Excellence
▶ National Performance Advisory Group
▶ NHS
▶ NHS Benchmarking Network
▶ NHS Clinical Commissioners
▶ NHS Confederation
▶ NHS Digital
▶ NHS Employers
▶ NHS England
▶ NHS Improvement
▶ NHS Leadership Academy
▶ NHS Providers
▶ NHS Resolution
▶ Nuffield Trust
▶ Professional Standards Authority
▶ Public Health England
▶ Skills for Care
▶ Social Care Institute for Excellence
▶ UK Government

47.2. STANDARDS

47.2.1. GOVERNANCE

LEGISLATION, STANDARDS AND FRAMEWORKS

▶ Relevant UK legislation
▶ Leadership Qualities Framework
▶ Manager Induction Standards
▶ NICE Quality Standards
▶ CQC Inspection Framework

GOVERNANCE DEFINITION

▶ Entirety of all systems and processes concerned with ensuring the overall direction, effectiveness, supervision and accountability of an organisation or service

GOVERNANCE CRITERIA

▶ Clear and traceable responsibility
▶ Informed and ethical leaders
  • Making it easier to do the right thing
  • Making it harder to do the wrong thing
▶ Alert and agile boards

47.2.2. CONDUCT

CONDUCT CODE FOR NHS MANAGERS

▶ Make the care and safety of patients your first concern and act to protect them from risk.
▶ Respect the public, patients, relatives, carers, staff and partners in other agencies.
▶ Be honest and act with integrity.
▶ Accept responsibility for your own work and the proper performance of the people you manage.

▶ Show your commitment to working as a team member by working with all your colleagues in the NHS and the wider community.

▶ Take responsibility for your own learning and development.

SEVEN PRINCIPLES OF PUBLIC LIFE

▶ Selflessness
▶ Integrity
▶ Objectivity
▶ Accountability
▶ Openness
▶ Honesty
▶ Leadership

SIX C'S OF HEALTHCARE EXCELLENCE

▶ Care
▶ Commitment
▶ Communication
▶ Compassion
▶ Competence
▶ Courage

47.3. INDUCTION

INDUCTION STANDARDS

▶ Core standards
  • Governance and accountability
  • Information and communication
  • Relationships and partnerships
  • Patient centred practice
  • Team oriented management
  • Finances and resources
  • Equality and diversity
  • Safeguarding and protection

▶ Optional standards
- Professional development
- Change management
- Business management
- Quality assurance

GOVERNANCE AND ACCOUNTABILITY

▶ Organisation
- Legislation
- Policies
- Governance structure
- Workplace culture

▶ Role
- Responsibility
- Accountability

▶ Environment
- Health
- Safety
- Risk management
- Infection prevention

▶ Challenges
- Concerns
- Complaints

INFORMATION AND COMMUNICATION

▶ Information management
▶ Confidentiality requirements
▶ Communication process

RELATIONSHIPS AND PARTNERSHIPS

▶ Collaborating
▶ Connecting
▶ Exchanging

▶ Linking

▶ Networking

▶ Socialising

PATIENT CENTRED PRACTICE

▶ Patient centred practice and outcome based practice
  - Patient centred practice
    - Personalised care
    - Coordinated care
    - Compassionate care
    - Dignified care
    - Enabling care
    - Respectful care
  - Outcome based practice
    - Morbidity levels
    - Mortality levels

▶ Patients' rights and patients' risks
  - Active participation
  - Choice
  - Control
  - Dignity
  - Independence
  - Individuality
  - Information
  - Needs
  - Preferences
  - Respect
  - Wishes
  - Risk taking

▶ Positive risk taking is weighing up the potential benefits and harms of choosing one action over another.
  - Risks cannot usually be eliminated altogether, but negligence can.

- Risks are seen not as danger, but as reward.

▶ Active participation and risk taking
  - Risk assessment
    - Clinical assessment
    - Actuarial assessment
  - Key questions
    - Can you justify your decisions with regard to the assessment of the patient?
    - Can you defend your decisions with regard to the assessment of the patient?

▶ Active participation and risk taking
  - Risk assessment
    - Collected all information?
    - Evaluated all risks?
    - Applied absolutely reliable methods?
    - Taken all reasonable steps?
    - Worked within the law?
    - Observed all policies?
    - Recorded all decisions?

TEAM ORIENTED MANAGEMENT

▶ Team management
▶ Team leadership
▶ Team vision
▶ Team development
▶ Team conflicts
▶ Team performance

▶ Team management implies a high level of concern for both the tasks and the people.
▶ Team management is an effective style with the potential for both high performance and happiness.

FINANCES AND RESOURCES

▶ Finances and contracts
▶ Resources and sustainability
▶ Recruitment and retention

EQUALITY AND DIVERSITY

▶ Equality
▶ Diversity
▶ Inclusion
▶ Discrimination

SAFEGUARDING AND PROTECTION

▶ Abuse and neglect
▶ Safeguarding and protection

PROFESSIONAL DEVELOPMENT

▶ Learning opportunities
▶ Development objectives
▶ Support
▶ Guidance
▶ Supervision practice
▶ Performance management

CHANGE MANAGEMENT

▶ Current market and service provision
▶ Change processes and service provision
▶ Growth of the organisation
▶ Sustainability of the organisation

BUSINESS MANAGEMENT

▶ Strategic management
▶ Operational management

QUALITY ASSURANCE

▶ Continuous quality improvement
  ● Quality standards
  ● Quality indicators
  ● Quality controls
▶ Culture of responsibility for quality
▶ Positive patient outcomes
  ● Best practice
  ● Improvement process
  ● Achievement measurement

MANAGEMENT PROCESS

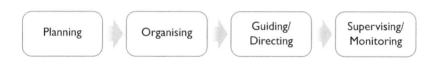

47.4. DEVELOPMENT

PROFESSIONAL DEVELOPMENT

▶ Dedicated time is critical to developing skills.
▶ Peer learning and peer support are essential.
▶ Shadowing opportunities are crucial for gaining experience.

▶ Principles for continuing professional development in healthcare
  ● Individual responsibility
    ▪ Identifying requirements
    ▪ Prioritising requirements

- - Learning
  - Recording
  - Scope of practice
  - Importance of reflection
  - Continuous appraisal

▶ Management of continuing professional development in a team
  - Regular supervision
  - Development plans
  - Formal learning
  - Reflective practice
  - Constructive feedback
  - Coaching approaches
  - Professional networks

▶ Different learning styles
  - Theoretical
  - Pragmatic
  - Intuitive
  - Reflective

▶ Personal development plan
  - Objectives
    - SMART: Specific, measurable, achievable, relevant, timed
  - Priorities
  - Activities
  - Resources and support
  - Barriers and blockers
  - Timeframe
  - Review
  - Outcome

▶ Reflective practice as a tool to improve performance
  - 360 degree reflection

▶ Topics for reflection as keys to learning
- Assessments
- Audits
- Claims
- Complaints
- Complications
- Compliments
- Discrepancies
- Errors
- Events
- Feedback
- Incidents

48 HEALTHCARE LEADERS

CHAPTER OVERVIEW

▶ LEADERS
- DEFINITIONS
  - MANAGERS
  - LEADERS
  - MANAGERS AND LEADERS
  - EXECUTIVES
- QUALITIES
  - LEADERSHIP QUALITIES FRAMEWORK
  - DIMENSIONS OF THE LEADERSHIP QUALITIES FRAMEWORK
  - DEMONSTRATING PERSONAL QUALITIES
  - WORKING WITH OTHERS
  - MANAGING SERVICES
  - IMPROVING SERVICES
  - SETTING DIRECTION
  - CREATING THE VISION
  - DELIVERING THE STRATEGY
- COMPETENCES
  - COMPETENCES
- PERSONALITY
  - PERSONALITY
- TRAITS
  - THE INDIVIDUAL
  - THE TEAM
  - THE PROCESS
  - THE RESULT
  - THE ASPIRATION
  - SUCCESSFUL TRAITS OF YESTERDAY'S LEADERS
  - SUCCESSFUL TRAITS OF TODAY'S LEADERS
  - TIMELESS TRAITS OF ALL LEADERS
- BEHAVIOURS
  - BEHAVIOURS
- CHALLENGES
  - DAILY CHALLENGES
  - PATIENT SAFETY
  - CARE QUALITY

- ■ **COMPELLING VISION**
- ■ **POWERFUL STRATEGY**
- ■ **HAVING SPACE**
- ■ **SOLVING PROBLEMS**
- ■ **REACHING HIGHER**
- ■ **LEADING TRANSPARENTLY**
- • **PARTICIPATION**
  - ■ **PHYSICIAN LEADERSHIP**
  - ■ **COLLECTIVE LEADERSHIP**

48.1. LEADERSHIP

48.1.1. PRINCIPLES

SYSTEM LEADERSHIP PRINCIPLES

▶ Behaving decently

▶ Behaving unselfishly

▶ Cultivating compassion

▶ Cultivating optimism

▶ Surfacing conflicts

▶ Surfacing problems

▶ Sharing purpose

▶ Sharing vision

▶ Communicating

▶ Inspiring

▶ Collaborating

▶ Integrating

▶ Developing trust

▶ Developing mutuality

▶ Forging cohesion

▶ Forging alliances

▶ Transforming relationships

▶ Transforming systems

▶ Rethinking radically
▶ Rethinking holistically

48.1.2. ELEMENTS

LEADERSHIP ELEMENTS

Leadership elements				
Leading self	Engaging others	Achieving results	Developing coalitions	Transforming systems

KEY ELEMENTS OF EFFECTIVE LEADERSHIP

▶ Authenticity
▶ Service orientation
▶ Emotional intelligence
  • Self awareness
  • Self management
  • Social awareness
  • Situational awareness
▶ Excellent communication
▶ Authority

▶ Clarity
▶ Consistency
▶ Commitment
▶ Courage
  • At all levels
  • At all times

▶ Driving for high performance
▶ Focusing on outstanding people

HOLISTIC APPROACH

▶ Leadership is not about a single person. Leadership is about many people at all levels sharing values, behaviours and goals. Leadership is about a truly holistic approach.

48.1.3. RESPONSIBILITIES

RESPONSIBILITIES

▶ Focusing on safe, high quality, truly compassionate and supportive care

▶ Ensuring direction, alignment and commitment of teams, services and organisations

▶ Aligning goals, values, ideas, thoughts, feelings and emotions

▶ Nurturing positive attitudes
▶ Sensing possible problems
▶ Improving organisational functioning
▶ Promoting staff participation
▶ Encouraging responsible innovation
▶ Engaging external stakeholders
▶ Developing cooperative relationships

DECISION MAKING

▶ Spectrum of decision making
  • Analysis
  • Integration
  • Intuition
▶ Obstacles to decision making
  • Too much information
  • Too much time
  • Too much emotion

▶ Consequences of decision making
  • Execution
  • Change
  • Accountability

48.1.4. IMPACT

IMPACT

▶ High quality leaders are the single most important factor in the success of any enterprise.

▶ High quality leaders are fundamental to the delivery of high quality care.

▶ High quality leaders are needed across all professions and at all levels.

▶ High quality leaders share leadership by working collaboratively.
  • They have inclusive and compassionate leadership skills.

▶ High quality leaders see what needs to be done and work with others to get it done.
  • They have executive and transformational leadership skills.

▶ High quality leaders work across all traditional boundaries in new care models – and not just from the board to the ward.
  • They have system and integration leadership skills.

▶ High quality leaders challenge the status quo, innovate, and inspire the future workforce.

▶ High quality leaders crack corporate concrete.

▶ High quality leaders are the most influential factor in shaping organisational culture at every level.

48.1.5. DEVELOPMENT

DEVELOPMENT

▶ Leadership is a precious resource in short supply.

▶ Achieving stronger leadership capacity
  - Increasing the quantity
  - Improving the quality

▶ Reading is important.
▶ Listening is more important.
▶ Practising is the most important.

▶ Leaders must understand how healthcare operates at the front line.

▶ Experience in leadership is the most valuable factor for the development of skills.
  - Extensive experience ranks higher than formal training.
  - Learning from experience should be a priority.

▶ Leadership is a lifelong learning and adapting experience.

▶ Leadership excellence requires international experience.

▶ High performing healthcare organisations are likely to have long serving senior leaders.

LEADERSHIP DEVELOPMENT ORGANISATIONS

▶ NHS Leadership Academy
▶ Faculty of Medical Leadership and Management
▶ Skills for Care

LEADERSHIP DEVELOPMENT INTERVENTIONS

▶ Multi-source feedback
▶ In-basket exercises
▶ Interviews
▶ Reflection
▶ Aptitude tests
▶ Group exercises

48.1.6. LEVELS

LEVELS

▶ Front-line worker
▶ Front-line leadership
▶ Operational leadership
▶ Strategic leadership

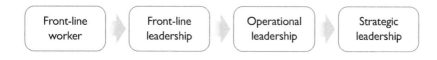

▶ Individual level
▶ Team level
▶ Board level
▶ National level

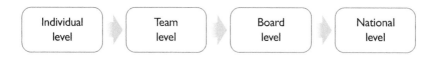

48.1.7. STYLES

LEADERSHIP STYLES

▶ Leadership is a process of influence towards the achievement of a goal.

▶ Different classifications based on different criteria
- Level of authority of leader
- Level of autonomy of team
- Personality of leader
- Purpose of leader

▶ Autocratic leadership
▶ Democratic leadership
▶ Consultative leadership
▶ Controlling leadership
▶ Enabling leadership

▶ People-oriented leadership
▶ Task-oriented leadership
▶ Target-oriented leadership
▶ Results-oriented leadership
▶ Action-oriented leadership

▶ Transactional leadership
▶ Transformational leadership

▶ Heroic leadership
▶ Charismatic leadership
▶ Bureaucratic leadership

- ▶ Ethical leadership
  - • Transformational leadership
  - • Value based leadership
  - • Servant leadership

- ▶ Collective leadership
  - • Everyone counts
  - • Everyone matters
  - • Everyone contributes
  - • Of all
  - • By all
  - • For all

- ▶ The leader's personality shapes the leadership style.
- ▶ The leadership style shapes the employees' behaviour, attitudes and function.
- ▶ The employees' behaviour, attitudes and function shape the service's performance.
- ▶ The service's performance shapes the organisation's future.

LEADERSHIP ACTIVITIES

- ▶ Advising
- ▶ Directing
- ▶ Controlling
- ▶ Collaborating
- ▶ Guiding
- ▶ Coordinating
- ▶ Participating
- ▶ Empowering
- ▶ Delegating

POWER TYPES

- ▶ Power through competence
- ▶ Power through position

▶ Power through reputation
▶ Power through respect
▶ Power through reward
▶ Power through punishment

POSITIVE LEADERSHIP STYLE

▶ Leadership is through trust – not through insecurity.
▶ Leadership is through influence – not through instruction.
▶ Leadership is through recommendation – not through imposition.
▶ Leadership is through negotiation – not through intimidation.

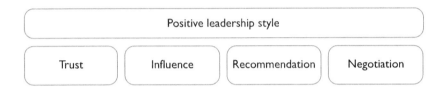

▶ Insecurity, instruction, imposition and intimidation never drive top level performance.

▶ Leadership is through authority of knowledge – not through authority of position.

▶ Natural authority comes from one who knows.
  • Natural authority attracts respect.
▶ Moral authority comes from enduring something together.
  • Moral authority attracts affection.

▶ Leadership is about working with individuals and teams – and earning their respect or even affection.
  • Trust is the essence of life.

▶ In leadership, example is everything: Leaders should model the standards and the behaviours they expect of their employees.

▶ Studies clearly demonstrate the value of authentic and transformational leadership as a predictor of quality outcomes in healthcare.

▶ Link between leadership and quality
  - Patient mortality
  - Patient satisfaction
  - Staff wellbeing
  - Staff morale
  - Staff engagement
  - Individual performance
  - Organisational performance

▶ Partnership between general and medical leaders is very important.

▶ Strong physician leadership is associated with improved organisational outcomes.

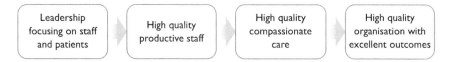

BEST LEADERSHIP STYLE

▶ Adjusted to the situation
▶ Adjusted to the people
  - The right style at the right time

Best leadership style	
Adjusted to the situation	Adjusted to the people

- ▶ Optimally balancing the task, individual and team
- ▶ Having maximum positive impact on other people
- ▶ Best fitting the organisation, vision and context

- ▶ Creating a positive vision
- ▶ Radiating a positive energy
- ▶ Projecting a positive optimism
- ▶ Promoting a positive culture

- ▶ Practising fairness
- ▶ Practising empathy
- ▶ Practising gratitude
- ▶ Practising generosity

- ▶ Excellent leadership has an incredible power.

48.1.8. CULTURE

LEADERSHIP CULTURE

- ▶ Championing leadership
- ▶ Developing leadership
- ▶ Practising leadership
- ▶ Rewarding leadership

ORGANISATIONAL CULTURE

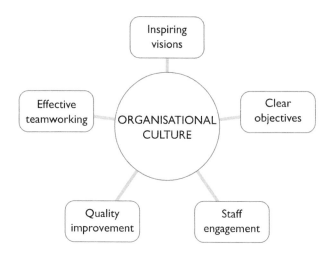

48.2. LEADERS

48.2.1. DEFINITIONS

MANAGERS

▶ Managers
- Administer
- Maintain
- Imitate
- Are reactive
- Request
- Instruct
- Push
- Accept the status quo
- Have knowledge
- Set the plan
- Plan details
- Ask how and when
- Focus on structures

- Have subordinates
- Control their staff
- Take a short term view
- Make decisions
- Make rules
- Avoid risks
- Desire results
- Do things right
- Take credit
- Attribute blame

LEADERS

▶ Leaders
- Innovate
- Change
- Originate
- Are proactive
- Empower
- Influence
- Pull
- Challenge the status quo
- Have wisdom
- Set the vision
- Set direction
- Ask what and why
- Focus on people
- Have followers
- Trust their staff
- Take a long term view
- Facilitate change
- Break rules
- Take risks
- Desire excellence
- Do the right thing
- Give credit
- Take blame

MANAGERS AND LEADERS

▶ Managers manage.
  • Managers have an assigned position.
▶ Leaders lead.
  • Leaders have an achieved position.

▶ Managers organise staff, leaders align people.
▶ Managers solve problems, leaders inspire people.
▶ Managers manage work, leaders lead people.

▶ Relationship between management and leadership
  • Perspective 1: Leadership alongside management
  • Perspective 2: Leadership overlapping with management
  • Perspective 3: Leadership within management

▶ The separation of management from leadership is harmful.
  • Management without leadership leads to discouragement and demotivation.
  • Leadership without management leads to disconnect and hubris.

▶ Management and leadership are distinct but complementary activities.

▶ The best executives are excellent at both activities.

▶ Healthcare organisations are very often over-managed but under-led.

EXECUTIVES

▶ Healthcare executives must be both managers and leaders.

▶ 'Knowing the right way'
▶ 'Going the right way'
▶ 'Showing the right way'

48.2.2. QUALITIES

LEADERSHIP QUALITIES FRAMEWORK

▶ Placing leadership at the very heart of social care
  • Five dimensions for all social care professionals
  • Two dimensions for most senior staff only

DIMENSIONS OF THE LEADERSHIP QUALITIES FRAMEWORK

▶ Demonstrating personal qualities
▶ Working with others
▶ Managing services
▶ Improving services
▶ Setting direction
▶ Creating the vision
  • For most senior staff only
▶ Delivering the strategy
  • For most senior staff only

DEMONSTRATING PERSONAL QUALITIES

▶ Developing self awareness
▶ Managing oneself effectively
▶ Continuing personal development
▶ Acting with integrity

WORKING WITH OTHERS

▶ Developing networks
▶ Building sustainable relationships
▶ Encouraging contribution
▶ Working within teams

MANAGING SERVICES

▶ Planning purposefully
▶ Managing resources
▶ Managing people
▶ Managing performance

IMPROVING SERVICES

▶ Ensuring safety
▶ Evaluating critically
▶ Encouraging innovation
▶ Facilitating transformation

SETTING DIRECTION

▶ Identifying contexts for change
▶ Applying knowledge and evidence
▶ Making decisions
▶ Evaluating impact

CREATING THE VISION

▶ Developing the vision
▶ Influencing the vision
▶ Communicating the vision
▶ Embodying the vision
▶ Reflecting the vision
  • Key characteristics of compelling visions
    ▪ Imaginable
    ▪ Desirable
    ▪ Feasible
    ▪ Focused
    ▪ Flexible
    ▪ Communicable

DELIVERING THE STRATEGY

▶ Framing the strategy
▶ Developing the strategy
▶ Implementing the strategy
▶ Embedding the strategy
▶ Reviewing the strategy

48.2.3. COMPETENCES

COMPETENCES

▶ Technical competence
   • Knowledge
▶ Conceptual competence
   • Understanding the complex internal and external environments of organisations
▶ Interpersonal competence
   • Emotions

▶ The competence level of a leader has a strong positive influence on the job satisfaction of an employee.

▶ Excellent leaders are expert leaders.

48.2.4. PERSONALITY

PERSONALITY

▶ Emotional maturity
▶ Determination
▶ Assertiveness
▶ High need for achievement
▶ Low need for affiliation

▶ High need for power
▶ Stamina
▶ Resilience
▶ Stress tolerance

▶ Being aware of own strengths
▶ Being aware of own typical reactions to situations
▶ Being aware of own limitations

▶ Social awareness

▶ Ability for
  ● Self-analysis
  ● Self-assessment
  ● Self-assurance
  ● Self-awareness
  ● Self-belief
  ● Self-confidence
  ● Self-control
  ● Self-determination
  ● Self-development
  ● Self-direction
  ● Self-esteem
  ● Self-evaluation
  ● Self-honesty
  ● Self-image
  ● Self-improvement
  ● Self-knowledge
  ● Self-management
  ● Self-mastery
  ● Self-questioning
  ● Self-reflection
  ● Self-regard
  ● Self-regulation

- Self-reliance
- Self-responsibility
- Self-restraint

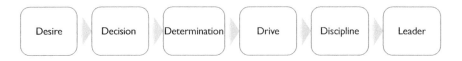

▶ Leaders continually monitor themselves, are never absolutely satisfied with their own performance and constantly question themselves.

▶ Successful leaders are a work-in-progress – adaptable, flexible and adjustable.

48.2.5. TRAITS

THE INDIVIDUAL

▶ One person can make a difference.

THE TEAM

▶ But when all persons share a common vision, together they can make an enormous difference.

THE PROCESS

▶ This is why each one of us should be fully committed to reaching further in every job we do.

THE RESULT

▶ None of us is as successful as all of us. Together, we reach further. A successful organisation is an interconnected group of successful teams.

THE ASPIRATION

▶ Striving for excellence
▶ Embracing change and innovation
▶ Championing top healthcare

SUCCESSFUL TRAITS OF YESTERDAY'S LEADERS

▶ Cognitive abilities
▶ Administrative skills
▶ Thoroughness
▶ Rigour

SUCCESSFUL TRAITS OF TODAY'S LEADERS

▶ Relationship building
▶ Communication skills
▶ Engagement
▶ Inspiration

TIMELESS TRAITS OF ALL LEADERS

▶ Ability
▶ Ambition

▶ Mindset skills
▶ Technical skills
▶ People skills
▶ Strategic skills
▶ Organisational skills
▶ Political skills

▶ Embracing the future
▶ Having high aspirations

▶ Having clear perspective
▶ Seeing possibilities
▶ Taking control
▶ Finding solutions
▶ Building momentum
▶ Creating great teams
▶ Creating good luck
▶ Focusing on execution

▶ Occasionally walking in front
▶ Sometimes walking beside
▶ Mostly walking behind
▶ Always walking with others

▶ Navigator
▶ Motivator
▶ Teacher
▶ Guide
▶ Coach
▶ Model

▶ Accessible
▶ Accountable
▶ Accurate
▶ Active
▶ Adaptable
▶ Agile
▶ Agreeable
▶ Ambitious
▶ Analytical
▶ Approachable
▶ Aspirational
▶ Assertive
▶ Attentive

- ▶ Authentic
- ▶ Calm
- ▶ Capable
- ▶ Caring
- ▶ Charismatic
- ▶ Cheerful
- ▶ Collaborative
- ▶ Committed
- ▶ Compassionate
- ▶ Compelling
- ▶ Competent
- ▶ Confident
- ▶ Conscientious
- ▶ Consistent
- ▶ Constructive
- ▶ Convincing
- ▶ Courageous
- ▶ Courteous
- ▶ Creative
- ▶ Credible
- ▶ Curious
- ▶ Decisive
- ▶ Dedicated
- ▶ Determined
- ▶ Diligent
- ▶ Diplomatic
- ▶ Disciplined
- ▶ Effective
- ▶ Empathetic
- ▶ Enabling
- ▶ Encouraging
- ▶ Energetic
- ▶ Enthusiastic
- ▶ Ethical
- ▶ Expert
- ▶ Extrovert

- ▶ Fair
- ▶ Flexible
- ▶ Focused
- ▶ Friendly
- ▶ Genuine
- ▶ Helpful
- ▶ Honest
- ▶ Hopeful
- ▶ Humble
- ▶ Humorous
- ▶ Inclusive
- ▶ Independent
- ▶ Influential
- ▶ Innovative
- ▶ Insistent
- ▶ Inspiring
- ▶ Intelligent
- ▶ Intuitive
- ▶ Kind
- ▶ Logical
- ▶ Loyal
- ▶ Mindful
- ▶ Open
- ▶ Optimistic
- ▶ Organised
- ▶ Passionate
- ▶ Perseverant
- ▶ Persistent
- ▶ Persuasive
- ▶ Polite
- ▶ Positive
- ▶ Pragmatic
- ▶ Proactive
- ▶ Productive
- ▶ Professional
- ▶ Proud

- ▶ Relentless
- ▶ Reliable
- ▶ Resilient
- ▶ Respectful
- ▶ Responsible
- ▶ Responsive
- ▶ Selfless
- ▶ Sensitive
- ▶ Sincere
- ▶ Skilled
- ▶ Straightforward
- ▶ Supportive
- ▶ Talented
- ▶ Thorough
- ▶ Tireless
- ▶ Tolerant
- ▶ Transparent
- ▶ Trusting
- ▶ Trustworthy
- ▶ Unstoppable
- ▶ Versatile
- ▶ Visible
- ▶ Visionary
- ▶ Warm
- ▶ Welcoming

48.2.6. BEHAVIOURS

BEHAVIOURS

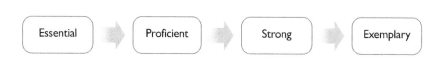

▶ Leading with care
▶ Sharing the vision
▶ Inspiring purpose
▶ Evaluating information
▶ Developing capability
▶ Engaging teams
▶ Connecting services
▶ Influencing for results
▶ Holding to account

▶ Interpreting the meaning of events
▶ Explaining the sense of change
▶ Creating an atmosphere of collective identity
▶ Encouraging commitment and optimism
▶ Building cohesion and trust

▶ Getting things right
▶ Making things better
  • Challenging beyond own remit
  • Caring beyond own remit
▶ Concern for excellence
▶ Attention to detail

▶ Making work better
  • Using 'Six Sigma'
    ▪ DMAIC: Define, measure, analyse, improve, control
▶ Making work faster
  • Using 'Lean Principles'

▶ Delighting patients
  • Better care
  • Faster care
▶ Working together
  • Better teamwork

▶ Using data
  ● Better decisions
▶ Improving processes
  ● Better flow
  ● Less variation

▶ All successful leaders have their own idiosyncrasies – and that is a good thing.

▶ Success = Great talent + high intelligence + hard work + good luck

48.2.7. CHALLENGES

DAILY CHALLENGES

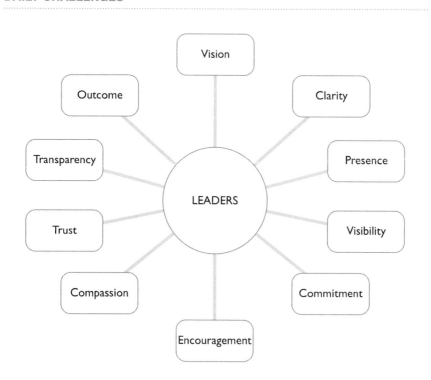

PATIENT SAFETY

▶ Leaders must always place the quality of care in general, and the safety of patients in particular, above all other aims.

CARE QUALITY

▶ Leaders must respond directly, openly and rapidly to patient complaints, early warnings and quality alerts.

COMPELLING VISION

▶ Leaders should have a purpose and vision and focus on pride and joy.

POWERFUL STRATEGY

▶ Leaders should forget about yesterday, live for today and plan for tomorrow.

HAVING SPACE

▶ Leaders need room to lead.

SOLVING PROBLEMS

▶ Leaders should train staff to bring solutions, not problems.
  • Any 'There is something wrong' should always be met with 'What should be done?'.
▶ Leaders should view themselves as catalysts for problem solving.

REACHING HIGHER

▶ Leaders should imagine the possibilities, accelerate the solutions and build the future.
  • The vision of a better future is a powerful motivating force.

LEADING TRANSPARENTLY

▶ Leaders must embrace transparency.

48.2.8. PARTICIPATION

PHYSICIAN LEADERSHIP

▶ Effective medical leadership is essential for excellence in healthcare and fundamental for transformation of healthcare.

▶ There is a strong correlation between physician leadership and organisational performance.

▶ Dimensions of medical leadership in healthcare
- Patients
- Doctors
- Other healthcare professionals
- Organisations
- Systems

▶ Role of medical leadership in healthcare
- Coordinating different professionals and leading across professional groups
- Driving change in organisations
  - Physician-led safety initiatives
  - Physician-led quality initiatives
- Impacting and influencing how organisations perform and improve

▶ Doctors becoming partners and shareholders
- Some power shifting from general managers to physician leaders and the front line, with benefits for patients and populations
  - Clinically led, management enabled
▶ Doctors accepting responsibility and accountability

COLLECTIVE LEADERSHIP

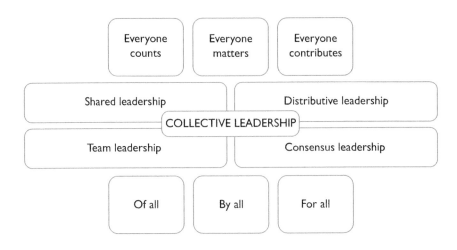

▶ Yesterday, power was held by the few.

▶ Today, power is made by the many.

▶ Collective leadership – as opposed to command-and-control structures – is characterised by shared leadership.

- The power is where the expertise is.
  - Shared thinking is stronger than solo thinking.
  - Shared thinking is more innovative than solo thinking.
  - Shared thinking is more productive than solo thinking.
  - Shared thinking is faster than solo thinking.
- Organisations should therefore build shared leadership capacity.

▶ Collective leadership – as opposed to command-and-control structures – requires that all employees matter.

▶ Collective leadership comes from anyone in the organisation and is focused on the achievement of a group rather than of an individual.

- Shared leadership actively supports team working.
- Shared leadership actively supports joint responsibility.

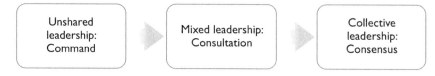

▶ Collective leadership is the optimum basis for caring cultures.

- All staff will ensure quality.
- All staff will intervene to solve problems.
- All staff will promote innovation.

▶ Collective leadership nurtures a corporate culture which delivers continually improving, high quality, truly compassionate care.

▶ Collective leadership accommodates the complexities of today's participative democratic environment in the best possible way.

49 HEALTHCARE EXECUTIVES

CHAPTER OVERVIEW

▶ EXECUTIVE RECRUITMENT
- LEADERSHIP GAPS
- BOARD VACANCIES
- DETERRING FACTORS
- SPECIFIC DISINCENTIVES
- ATTRACTING EXECUTIVES
- RETAINING EXECUTIVES

▶ GENERAL TIPS
- CAREER
  - TIPS FOR EXECUTIVES
- QUALITIES
  - TIPS FOR EXECUTIVES
- AGILITY
  - TIPS FOR EXECUTIVES
- ORGANISATION
  - TIPS FOR EXECUTIVES
- PEERS
  - TIPS FOR EXECUTIVES
- STAFF
  - TIPS FOR EXECUTIVES
- COMMUNICATION
  - TIPS FOR EXECUTIVES
- PRIORITISATION
  - TIPS FOR EXECUTIVES
- DECISION
  - TIPS FOR EXECUTIVES

- EXECUTION
  - TIPS FOR EXECUTIVES
- FEEDBACK
  - TIPS FOR EXECUTIVES
- CRITICISM
  - TIPS FOR EXECUTIVES
- COURAGE
  - TIPS FOR EXECUTIVES
- CHANGE
  - TIPS FOR EXECUTIVES
- UNCERTAINTY
  - TIPS FOR EXECUTIVES
- CRISIS
  - TIPS FOR EXECUTIVES
- MEDIA
  - TIPS FOR EXECUTIVES
- HAPPINESS
  - TIPS FOR EXECUTIVES

▶ BOARD CHAIR
- ROLE
  - ROLE
- QUALIFICATION
  - CAPABILITIES AND QUALITIES
  - KEY SUCCESS FACTORS
- RESPONSIBILITIES
  - KEY RESULT AREAS
  - MAIN FOCUS AREAS
- TIPS
  - TIPS FOR BOARD CHAIRS

▶ CHIEF EXECUTIVE
- ROLE
  - ROLE
- QUALIFICATION
  - CAPABILITIES AND QUALITIES
  - KEY SKILLS
  - KEY ATTRIBUTES

343

- RESPONSIBILITIES
  - KEY RESULT AREAS
  - OTHER MAJOR RESPONSIBILITIES
- TIPS
  - TIPS FOR CHIEF EXECUTIVES
▶ MEDICAL DIRECTOR
- ROLE
  - ROLE
- QUALIFICATION
  - CAPABILITIES AND QUALITIES
  - KEY SKILL AREAS
  - STRONG LEARNING CULTURE
  - STRONG IMPROVEMENT METHODOLOGY
  - KEY SUCCESS FACTORS
  - JOB DESCRIPTION
  - ADDITIONAL INFORMATION
  - PERSON SPECIFICATION
  - SAMPLE PROFILE
  - PROFESSIONAL SUPPORT
  - STAFF SUPPORT
  - OTHER ESSENTIALS
- RESPONSIBILITIES
  - KEY RESULT AREAS
  - OTHER MAJOR RESPONSIBILITIES
  - COMPLEX ORGANISATIONAL COMMITMENT
  - ENSURING CORPORATE PERFORMANCE
  - DEVELOPMENTAL PRIORITIES
  - OPERATIONAL PRIORITIES
  - RESPONSIBILITY AND ACCOUNTABILITY
  - RESPONSIBLE OFFICER'S ROLE
  - RESPONSIBLE CONSULTANT'S ROLE
  - APPRAISAL AND REVALIDATION
  - MENTORING DOCTORS
  - WRITING REFERENCES
- TIPS
  - TIPS FOR MEDICAL DIRECTORS

49.1. EXECUTIVE RECRUITMENT

LEADERSHIP GAPS

▶ Main reasons for leadership gaps
- Absence of talent management
- Absence of leadership development
- Absence of recruitment strategy
- Absence of succession planning
- Absence of attractive conditions

BOARD VACANCIES

▶ Negative impact of board level vacancies on a healthcare organisation
- Strategic instability
- Operational instability
- Low staff morale
- Low staff engagement
- High costs
- Low performance

DETERRING FACTORS

▶ Main deterring factors for board level positions
- Excessive regulation
- High workload
- Limited autonomy
- Frequent inspections
- Unrealistic expectations
- Media awareness
- Public scrutiny
- Blame culture
- Personal exposure
- Instant accountability
- Disproportionate consequences
- Structural uncertainties

- Redundancy terms
- Short tenure
- Inadequate pay

▶ Main deterring factors for Medical Director positions
- Formal clinical accountabilities
  - Responsible Officer role
  - Clinical workforce representation role
  - Caldicott Guardian role
- Unattractive risk-reward ratio
- Unattractive work-life balance
- Low peer support

SPECIFIC DISINCENTIVES

▶ Main specific disincentives for Medical Director positions
- Loss of clinical experience
- Loss of clinical credibility
- Perceived job insecurity
- Limited financial incentives

ATTRACTING EXECUTIVES

▶ Executive positions: 'Moving to the dark side'?

▶ The job needs to be more enticing, more manageable, more sustainable and more valued.

▶ The tenure needs to last long enough to build relationships, change culture, deliver results and increase performance.

▶ Medical clinician: 'The flawless doctor'?
▶ Medical Director: 'The grubby businessman'?

- ▶ Ending the disgraceful denigration of clinical leaders
    - Politics and media
- ▶ Ending the restraint on reward
    - 'You get what you pay for …'
- ▶ Ending the double jeopardy for clinical leaders
    - NHS and GMC

- ▶ Doctors appointed to leadership positions, e.g. Medical Director, should be allowed to return to their previous position, e.g. Consultant, at the end of their term of appointment.

RETAINING EXECUTIVES

- ▶ Shining light on the 'dark side'
- ▶ Eradicating the 'them and us' attitude
- ▶ Shifting executives to the 'enlightened side'

- ▶ Leadership excellence should be valued across all disciplines and all levels.

49.2. GENERAL TIPS

49.2.1. CAREER

TIPS FOR EXECUTIVES

✓ Do not expect Human Resources to plan your career.

✓ Your destiny is your responsibility.
✓ Be goal driven: Know what to do next.
✓ Your destiny determines your legacy.

✓ Build your career.
    - Assess your skills.

- Fill your gaps.
- Broaden your horizons.
- Step out of your comfort zone and expand your world.
- Check your market value.
- Switch your radar on.
- Give it a go.

✓ You should be relentlessly driven by possibilities.
  - You are always on a learning curve.
✓ You should be enthusiastic about the future.

✓ You can be immensely proud of being appointed to one of the most senior leadership roles.
  - Express your gratitude.
  - Convey your appreciation.
  - Celebrate your success.

49.2.2. QUALITIES

TIPS FOR EXECUTIVES

✓ Be mindful of essential attributes of an executive, such as integrity, practical wisdom, moral authority and humility.
  - Integrity requires truthfulness, incorruptibility and candour.
  - Practical wisdom requires aptitude, practice and reflection.
  - Moral authority requires honesty, fairness and modesty.
  - Humility requires respectfulness, courtesy and unpretentiousness.

✓ Mindfulness means being alert, attentive and aware.
✓ Mindfulness means being conscious, creative and compassionate.
✓ Mindfulness means living in the moment.
✓ Mindfulness means less stress, worry and pessimism.
✓ Mindfulness means better focus, work and health.

✓ Shake up your daily routine to gain perspective, reorient yourself and increase concentration.

....

✓ Assess yourself before you assess others.
✓ Do not overestimate your strengths.
✓ Do not underestimate your weaknesses.
✓ Beware of too much introspection, though.

....

✓ It is all about how you are – and how you come across.

....

✓ Do not emulate others.
✓ Do not copy others.
✓ Be genuine.
✓ Be yourself.
✓ Show your unique qualities.
✓ Develop your personal brand.

....

✓ Live your brand.

....

✓ Manage your time.
✓ Maximise your strengths.
✓ Overcome your blind spots.
  • Leverage your relationships to complement your traits and to overcome your limitations.
✓ Delegate your weaknesses.
✓ Refine your brand.

....

✓ Personify and exemplify the qualities required and expected in your organisation.

....

✓ Minimise yourself, maximise your vision.

....

✓ Be honest.
  - Say what the truth is.
  - Say what you really mean.
✓ Be straight.
  - Observe the 'no hidden surprises' rule.
    - When needed, drive home uncomfortable messages.
✓ Be credible.
  - Do not oversell good news.
  - Do not undersell bad news.

✓ Liars will not be believed even when they speak the truth.

✓ Be transparent in all your actions.
✓ Be familiar with the rules and regulations about information disclosure.
✓ If in doubt, seek legal advice.

✓ The positive mood of an executive is infectious.
✓ The fervent emotions of an executive are contagious.

✓ Choose to make today a great day.
  - The staff's mood reflects your own mood.

✓ Smile.
✓ Accentuate the positive.
✓ Celebrate.

✓ Dress properly.
  - A little vanity is a good thing.
✓ Look smart.

✓ There is, however, a line between self-esteem and narcissism: Do not cross that line.

✓ Lead by walking around, getting around, being around.
- Listen.
- Communicate.
  - Effective communication is essential to positive relationships.
- Praise.

....

✓ A universal leader excels in human qualities such as fairness, goodness, humaneness, kindness and firmness.

49.2.3. AGILITY

TIPS FOR EXECUTIVES
....

✓ Do not be entrenched in your silo bubble.

....

✓ Avoid pigeonholing.
- There is always more than one perspective.

✓ Value difference.

....

✓ Stay mentally flexible.
✓ Step outside your boundaries.
✓ Always look outwards.

....

✓ Stretch your mind in different directions.
✓ Use lateral thinking.
✓ Analyse an issue from the point of view of someone else.
✓ Make creative connections.
✓ Develop a culture for breakthrough ideas.

....

✓ Conquer complacency and conformism. There is no place for complacency and conformism in healthcare. Complacency and conformism kill.

....

✓ Go beyond the obvious.

✓ If you can dream it, you can achieve it.

✓ Reach for the sky.

....

✓ Dream big, think differently, work better and become more.

....

✓ Big dreams bring big moves.

49.2.4. ORGANISATION

TIPS FOR EXECUTIVES

....

✓ You are the face of the organisation.

✓ Be outspoken in your praise for the organisation, wherever it is true.

✓ You are the ambassador of the organisation.

....

✓ Stand up for your organisation.
  • Broaden your mind.
  • Overcome mental blocks.
  • Challenge your assumptions.
  • Bring fresh thinking.
  • Encourage open dialogue.
  • Make a difference.

....

✓ Be positive about your organisation.

✓ Be positive about your vision.

✓ Be positive about your team.

✓ Be positive about your future.

....

✓ Reflect on your vision, discuss your vision and act upon your vision.
  • Leadership is about doing: Only vision with action can change the organisation.

....

✓ Do not disclose doubts, uncertainties, insecurities or worries about the future.

....

✓ Keep your goals, principles and values in mind.
✓ Make time for strategic planning.
✓ Change the direction when the situation demands it.

....

✓ A positive error culture is the key for creativity, innovation, risk taking and entrepreneurial acumen.
✓ There is no creativity, innovation, risk taking and entrepreneurial acumen without a positive error culture.

....

✓ Your office should be tidy, functional, technically well equipped, pleasant and comfortable.
  • Avoid ostentatious, flamboyant and luxurious equipment.

49.2.5. PEERS

TIPS FOR EXECUTIVES
....

✓ Know how things are done around here.
✓ Know who makes the running.
✓ Know what is going on behind the scenes.
✓ Know about any hidden agendas.
✓ Know strategies to deal with office politics.

....

✓ Surround yourself with great people.
✓ Ask these people for their advice.
✓ Meet people with similar minds.

....

✓ Identify reliable confidants.
✓ Develop relationships with those from varied backgrounds.
✓ Network with stakeholders.

....

✓ Do not force contacts: Your personal interests must coincide with your allies' interests.

✓ Develop allies and not mates.
✓ Keep a clear distinction between a working and a friendship relationship.
✓ Be friendly without being familiar.

✓ Do not confuse friendship with trust.

✓ Familiarity breeds contempt.
✓ A respectful distance is beneficial for the whole organisation.
  • Gravitas and charisma require a bit of aloofness.
✓ Proximity diminishes respect.

✓ Study the naysayers, opponents and rivals in your organisation.

✓ Also keep a wary eye on the 'yeasayers' who only bring good news.

49.2.6. STAFF

TIPS FOR EXECUTIVES

✓ Have respect for superiors, peers, subordinates – and yourself.

✓ The golden rule: Treat others as you would like to be treated.

✓ Value loyalty.
✓ Value intelligence.
✓ Value initiative.
✓ Value ambition.
✓ Value reliability.

✓ Beware of disloyalty.
✓ Beware of egoism.
✓ Beware of unprofessionalism.
✓ Beware of bravado.
✓ Beware of unreliability.

✓ Do not manage people – encourage them, facilitate them, empower them.

✓ Empower other people to shine.

✓ Acknowledge, compliment and praise others, including in public.

49.2.7. COMMUNICATION

TIPS FOR EXECUTIVES

✓ Listening proves that you value others.

✓ Listening provides insights, trains intuition and adds value.

✓ Listen to patients, staff and stakeholders.
✓ Read between the lines and understand the context.
✓ Observe, absorb and connect the circumstances.

✓ The importance of the interaction between individuals at board level and individuals at the front line cannot be overestimated.

✓ Walk the wards. Walk the offices. Walk the halls. Meet. Mingle. Merge.

✓ Facilitate conversations.

✓ Socialise actively.

✓ Make links.

✓ Form relationships.

✓ Work together.

✓ Share success.

✓ Communication is a complex process.

✓ Handle negative, aggressive and hostile people with kindness.

✓ Treat all people with respect.

✓ Be professional at all times.

✓ Manage your emotions.

✓ Do not raise your voice.

✓ Control your spoken word.

✓ Control your voice.

✓ Control your body language.

✓ Do not respond in or to anger. Let the anger remain with other people. Do not give anybody the 'evil eye'.

✓ Never write a message that degrades or belittles.

✓ Never write a message that is cynical or sarcastic.

✓ Spend your energy on positive thoughts and actions.

✓ Do not talk about others, because people assume that if you are talking to them about others, you are also talking to others about them.

✓ Stay away from gossip, alehouse politics and doubletalk.

✓ Never run down your employees behind their backs.

49.2.8. PRIORITISATION

TIPS FOR EXECUTIVES

✓ Focus on the pressing problems of the organisation.

✓ Prioritise your tasks.
  - Things you have to do …
  - Things you will do …
  - Things you would like to do …
  - Things you will not be able to do …
✓ Avoid time stealers, distractions, interruptions and idle talk.
✓ Organise your time.

✓ If you fail to plan, you plan to fail.

✓ Concentrate your forces.

49.2.9. DECISION

TIPS FOR EXECUTIVES

✓ Organisations are primarily seeking rigorous direction, not compliant oversight.

✓ People want to hear about solutions, not about problems.
  - You need problem solving skills.
  - You need decision making abilities.

✓ Listen empathetically.
✓ Consult your team.
✓ Analyse the issue.
✓ Do not rush.

✓ Respect different perspectives.

✓ Decide on facts.

✓ Communicate effectively.

....

✓ Always get various perspectives. Learn by putting the same question to different people. You will be amazed.

....

✓ Information should be checked.

✓ Facts should be contested.

✓ Views should be challenged.

✓ Emotions should be questioned.

....

✓ Narrow the gap between what people are thinking and what people are saying to bring the truth to the surface – and strive against dishonesty, mendacity, duplicity and hypocrisy.

....

✓ Have a clear timeframe for every decision.

✓ A wrong decision is better than no decision.

  • In each case, you make a decision with what you know at that moment.

✓ Grow your ability as a problem solver.

....

✓ Set clear deadlines, insist on regular progress reports and focus on results.

....

✓ You are judged both by the decisions you make and by the way you execute them: Make decisions and provide direction.

  • Bear in mind that informed, carefully thought out, collective decisions are the best decisions.

....

✓ Indecision kills morale, teams, projects and organisations.

....

✓ If your decision involves risks, analyse these for probability and impact.

....

✓ Think through the consequences of your decision – for your organisation, for your employees and for yourself.

....

✓ Seize the moment when the time is right for a decision.

....

✓ Do not withhold the rationale behind your decision.

....

✓ Do not make a decision against your better judgement.

....

✓ Communicate your decision to all those who will be affected.

....

✓ Amend your previous decision if, after consideration, you feel that the previous decision was wrong.

....

✓ Apologise when you have made a mistake.

49.2.10. EXECUTION

TIPS FOR EXECUTIVES

✓ Do things.
✓ Lead through actions, not words.
✓ Create value.

....

✓ Always do what you promise you will do – and in a timely manner.
  • Do not fall prey to the 'say-do gap'.

....

✓ Do more than wanted, better than needed and sooner than expected: You are the role model for your organisation.

49.2.11. FEEDBACK

TIPS FOR EXECUTIVES

✓ You cannot grow without feedback.
  - However, you do not need feedback from people who you know are mean-spirited.
✓ Take advantage of honest feedback.

49.2.12. CRITICISM

TIPS FOR EXECUTIVES

✓ Do not be afraid of criticism: Criticism makes you sharper and tougher.
  - But: You do have the right to choose your critics.
  - And: Do not listen to the first that comes along.
✓ Do not be afraid of failure: Failure helps you learn your lessons.

✓ Show strong political acumen.
✓ Solve controversial issues without having major disagreements, at least publicly.
✓ Do not shy away.

✓ Embrace constructive conflict.
✓ Convince with knowledge, arguments, kindness and inclusiveness.
✓ Persuade the unpersuaded.

✓ Live with setbacks.
✓ Learn from success, criticism and failure.
✓ Cope with disappointment.

✓ Appear strong under high pressure – even if you are not.

49.2.13. COURAGE

TIPS FOR EXECUTIVES

✓ Never hide yourself.
✓ Never turn a blind eye.
✓ Never avoid a difficult message.
✓ Never shy away.

✓ Embrace discomfort.

✓ Do not hide problems, because severe problems always surface.

✓ Remain courageous, fearless and confident even in the face of disapproval, criticism, rejection, opposition, setback and failure.

✓ Do the right thing – even when it is risky to do so.

✓ Never do what is easiest when you know it is not what is best.
  • Never follow the line of least resistance.
  • You need to forge ahead through adversity.

✓ Ignore the herd.
✓ Swim upstream.
✓ Avoid groupthink.
✓ Stand out.
✓ Gain an edge.

✓ Fortune favours the brave.

✓ Nothing should surprise you.
✓ Nothing should baffle you.

✓ Nothing should scare you.

✓ Acknowledge your fears – and conquer them.

✓ Hold to principles and ethics in tough times and under pressure.

✓ Stand for something.
✓ Be authentic.
✓ Be the type of person you want to be.
✓ Be clear.
✓ Never compromise values.

✓ Never give up: What you lose on the swings you gain on the roundabouts.

49.2.14. CHANGE

TIPS FOR EXECUTIVES

✓ Change is the best way to improve performance.

✓ Change requires
  • Good planning
  • Sensitivity
  • Reassurance for employees
  • Firmness
  • Strong leadership

✓ Start where you are.
✓ Use what you have.
✓ Do what you can.

✓ Push the boundaries, make things happen.

49.2.15. UNCERTAINTY

TIPS FOR EXECUTIVES

✓ Stay on track.
✓ Deal with events as they come.
✓ Focus on communication, prioritisation, task setting, team working, transparency and clarity.
✓ Be true to yourself and decide.
✓ Act with respect.

✓ Scenario planning and contingency planning mitigate the risks of uncertainty and chaos.

✓ Uncertainty and chaos bring discomfort and unease but also creativity and innovation.

49.2.16. CRISIS

TIPS FOR EXECUTIVES

✓ In a crisis, gather the facts.
✓ Analyse the situation.
✓ Specify the objectives.
✓ Set up a crisis management team.
✓ Line up a crisis management plan.
✓ Consider different actions.
✓ Evaluate possible alternatives.
✓ In a crisis, focus on communication.

✓ In every crisis there is an opportunity.
✓ Maintain a positive mood during downsizing and reconfiguration.
✓ Use budget cuts and financial restraints to review your hospital strategy and vision.

✓ Reallocate revenues to improve financial and operational performance.
✓ Effective communication is paramount during a crisis.

....

✓ In a crisis, lead from your head as well as from your heart.
  • Lead with confidence in your abilities.
  • Lead with strong teams.
  • Lead with courage, compassion and creativity.
  • Lead with genuine feelings.
  • Lead with persistence to a solution.
✓ In a crisis, true leaders stand out and live up to high expectations.

....

✓ Decide.
✓ Implement.
✓ Monitor.
✓ Re-evaluate.
✓ Communicate.

49.2.17. MEDIA

TIPS FOR EXECUTIVES

✓ Be prepared to say something, anywhere, anytime.
✓ Communicate promptly, transparently, purposefully, on a regular but also on an impromptu basis, to the relevant audiences, through the major media and across the right channels.
  • Be aware of unplanned, unexpected and unforeseen circumstances.
✓ Make sure you are proactive, positive, precise.

....

✓ What is your audience?
✓ What is your message?
  • Use simple, clear messages.
  • Back up with accurate, reliable evidence.
  • Use simple, plain language.
✓ What is your aim?

....

✓ Be open.

✓ Be truthful.

✓ Be friendly.

....

✓ Express your views comprehensibly, coherently and convincingly.

....

✓ Keep your communication short, simple, systematic and structured.

....

✓ Repeat key messages several times.

....

✓ Keep things as basic as possible.

49.2.18. HAPPINESS

TIPS FOR EXECUTIVES

✓ Look after yourself.

✓ Establish a support network outside your organisation and talk things through.

✓ Stay well connected.

....

✓ Protect your time.

✓ Protect your resilience.

✓ Protect your reputation.

✓ Protect your legacy.

....

✓ Do not deplete yourself.

✓ Always restore perspective and see the wider meaning in what you do.

  • Do not get down into the weeds.

✓ Plan your time off.

....

✓ Life is very short.

✓ Happiness in life is about love, optimism, self-determination, self-confidence, achievement and fulfilment.

✓ Do not waste time.

....

✓ Embark on a leadership journey which will take you wherever you aspire to go.

....

✓ Grab your opportunities.

✓ Take your chances.

✓ Appreciate your achievements.

....

✓ Celebrate success.

✓ Reward yourself.

✓ Take pride.

....

✓ Sit back, relax and pat yourself on the back for a job well done. You deserve it.

....

✓ Your job is fulfilling and energising, it is a privilege and an honour. Enjoy it.

49.3. BOARD CHAIR

49.3.1. ROLE

ROLE

▶ Board leadership

▶ Board building

▶ Board information

▶ Board communication

▶ Board cooperation

▶ Board evaluation

49.3.2. QUALIFICATION

CAPABILITIES AND QUALITIES

▶ Breaking down barriers
▶ Building new bridges
▶ Navigating their way carefully
▶ Adapting their approach to the people and circumstances
▶ Taking stakeholders with them
▶ Developing board members
▶ Leading by example

KEY SUCCESS FACTORS

▶ Relationship building
▶ Partnership working
▶ Leadership ability
▶ Strategic insight
▶ Boardroom competence

49.3.3. RESPONSIBILITIES

KEY RESULT AREAS

▶ Formulating strategy
▶ Shaping the culture
▶ Ensuring accountability

MAIN FOCUS AREAS

▶ Safe care
▶ Patient-centred care
▶ Partnership working between clinicians and managers
▶ Positive culture for risk management
  • Assurance processes with regard to safety and quality concerns

▶ Strong cooperation with GPs and community
▶ Forward-looking organisation
▶ Sustainable organisation

49.3.4. TIPS

TIPS FOR BOARD CHAIRS

✓ Your relationship with the Chief Executive is key to success.

✓ But: Remember that you are not the Chief Executive.
✓ And: You lead the board and not the organisation.
  • You are an important facilitator, but not the commander.

✓ Leave room for other people.
✓ Do not dominate.
✓ Restrain yourself.
✓ Do not rush.
✓ Encourage thoughtfulness and self reflection.

✓ Take board meetings seriously.
✓ Listen rather than speak.
  • Reduce your airtime to a minimum.
✓ Enable the board members.
✓ Remain unbiased and impartial.

✓ Plan board meetings properly.
  • Keep the topics on the agenda to a minimum.
  • Keep the presentations during the meeting to a minimum.
  • Keep the length of the meeting to a minimum.

✓ Take advantage of the diversity of backgrounds and sectors, of perspectives and visions, and of competence and experience within your organisation.

✓ Adopt a collective, shared, collaborative and inclusive style.
  - The all-knowing hero has gone, and so has the pace-setting approach.

✓ Create conditions under which board members can have productive discussions.

✓ Build a culture of candour, trust and openness.

✓ What matters most is your tenacity, curiosity, courage, communication and resilience.
  - Courage, in this context, means strength and agility.

✓ Learn to cope with adversity, stress and hostility.

49.4. CHIEF EXECUTIVE

49.4.1. ROLE

ROLE

▶ Top administrator of a healthcare organisation

▶ The role of Chief Executives in healthcare has never been more important than it is today.
  - They provide overall direction for the organisation within guidelines set up by the board.
  - They ensure that almost every aspect of how the organisation performs is working efficiently.

369

49.4.2. QUALIFICATION

CAPABILITIES AND QUALITIES

▶ Chief Executives should have proven senior level experience in complex political, financial and strategic environments within healthcare.

▶ Chief Executives should have an in-depth knowledge of local health services, of local, regional and central government structures, and of key policy makers.

▶ Chief Executives should have a deep understanding of the full capital investment cycle, from planning to commissioning, including the ability to analyse and interpret quantitative and qualitative information and data.

▶ Chief Executives should have a track record of creating strategies, interventions and innovative solutions to complex issues.

▶ Chief Executives should be able to build sustainable relations with partners, even in difficult circumstances.

▶ Chief Executives should have a commercial mindset.

KEY SKILLS

▶ Communicating effectively
▶ Embodying the common vision
▶ Creating a sense of purpose
▶ Coping with uncertainty
▶ Leading turnaround in distressed organisations
▶ Staying on track
▶ Setting a framework for success
▶ Adjusting the leadership style
▶ Thinking positively

KEY ATTRIBUTES

- ▶ Accountability
- ▶ Adaptability
- ▶ Agility
- ▶ Alertness
- ▶ Attentiveness
- ▶ Authenticity
- ▶ Awareness
- ▶ Character
- ▶ Charisma
- ▶ Charity
- ▶ Commitment
- ▶ Compassion
- ▶ Compatibility
- ▶ Competence
- ▶ Confidence
- ▶ Cooperativeness
- ▶ Courage
- ▶ Creativity
- ▶ Credibility
- ▶ Curiosity
- ▶ Decisiveness
- ▶ Dedication
- ▶ Deference
- ▶ Determination
- ▶ Diplomacy
- ▶ Discernment
- ▶ Discipline
- ▶ Drive
- ▶ Empathy
- ▶ Endurance
- ▶ Energy
- ▶ Enthusiasm
- ▶ Excellence
- ▶ Fairness

- ▶ Fearlessness
- ▶ Focus
- ▶ Foresight
- ▶ Forgiveness
- ▶ Generosity
- ▶ Gratitude
- ▶ Grit
- ▶ Honesty
- ▶ Humility
- ▶ Humour
- ▶ Impartiality
- ▶ Inclusiveness
- ▶ Independence
- ▶ Industriousness
- ▶ Initiative
- ▶ Insight
- ▶ Inspiration
- ▶ Instinct
- ▶ Integrity
- ▶ Judgement
- ▶ Kindness
- ▶ Knowledge
- ▶ Leadership
- ▶ Loyalty
- ▶ Magnetism
- ▶ Morality
- ▶ Openness
- ▶ Optimism
- ▶ Outspokenness
- ▶ Passion
- ▶ Perseverance
- ▶ Persistence
- ▶ Proactivity
- ▶ Probity
- ▶ Professionalism
- ▶ Reliability

- Resilience
- Respect
- Responsibility
- Responsiveness
- Sensitivity
- Sincerity
- Stamina
- Tact
- Teachability
- Toughness
- Transparency
- Trustworthiness
- Truthfulness
- Veracity
- Vision
- Wisdom
- Zest

49.4.3. RESPONSIBILITIES

KEY RESULT AREAS

- Statutory obligations
- Service obligations
- Overall accountability for the quality of patient care
- Managerial responsibility
- Financial responsibility

OTHER MAJOR RESPONSIBILITIES

- Producing project plans
- Engaging with key stakeholders
- Researching information, analysing data and presenting findings
- Developing recommendations for action

▶ Determining strategic change

▶ Undertaking option appraisals

▶ Performing thorough risk assessments

▶ Preparing documentation, managing procurement and influencing relationships

▶ Working with approving bodies

▶ Delivering positive outcomes

▶ Implementing new models of care

▶ Working collaboratively with partner organisations

▶ Meeting increasing demand with finite resources

▶ Adhering to strict financial controls

▶ Maintaining fit for purpose facilities

49.4.4. TIPS

TIPS FOR CHIEF EXECUTIVES

✓ Patient care must be your prime concern. Always!

✓ Maintain an overall focus on patient care. Always!

✓ You must know the weakest points of your organisation from the outset. Only then can you change and improve things at an early stage.

✓ You are the game changer in your organisation.
- Bring your experience to life with imagination.
- See possibilities where others see limits.
- Put your potential and ideas into practice.

✓ Challenge current practice and embrace prudent innovation.

✓ Transformational change requires strong leadership.
- Embody purpose.

- Inspire possibility.
- Create change.

....

✓ You can outperform your competitors with a strong focus on care quality, workplace attractiveness and high performance.

....

✓ Think beyond your current organisational boundaries.
✓ See the bigger picture.
✓ Spread your success to other organisations.

....

✓ Raise the bar. Aim high. Raise the altitude.

....

✓ Find clever ways around obstacles. Push hard, if necessary. But avoid the activity trap.

....

✓ Expect the most from yourself.

....

✓ With confidence you can go anywhere.

....

✓ Absolute integrity is one of the most important qualities of a Chief Executive: Integrity is a stepping stone towards trust.

....

✓ Never compromise your integrity.

....

✓ Provide governance.
✓ Comply with legal and ethical frameworks.
✓ Set boundaries.

....

✓ Make sure you have robust governance processes in place.
  - Formal arrangements
  - Consistent policies
  - Clear procedures

- Systematic monitoring
- Effective oversight

✓ Make sure you have effective risk assessment in place.
- Safety culture
- Clinical audit
- Incident reporting
- Benchmarking outcomes
- Learning culture

✓ You must act impartially.

✓ You must not be influenced by social, business or other relationships.

✓ You must decide transparently.

✓ You must declare all relevant interests.

✓ Rely on your purpose.

✓ Rely on your vision.

✓ Rely on your strategy.

✓ Rely on your employees.

✓ Rely on your strength.

✓ Develop your self awareness.

✓ Improve your listening skills.

✓ Be interested in others.

✓ Walk in others' shoes.

✓ Show your honest appreciation.

✓ Ensure your employees feel valued, encouraged, motivated and supported.

✓ Emotional intelligence is the *conditio sine qua non* of excellent leadership.

✓ Build emotional intelligence.
- Perceive and manage your own emotions and the emotions of others. This is not a nicety, this is a necessity.

✓ There is a strong link between emotional intelligence and leadership performance.

....

✓ Emotions can be harnessed, emotions can be integrated into thought, emotions can be applied to tasks, emotions can be regulated.

✓ Hence, you can motivate or demotivate, cheer up or calm down, move up or move down, hearten or dishearten others.

....

✓ Make use of your emotional intelligence.

....

✓ Leadership needs followership. Win the hearts and minds of your team. Never walk alone.

....

✓ Make your leadership visible.
  • Get out of your office and talk to patients, staff, partners and stakeholders.
✓ Explain your leadership policy.

....

✓ You are the cheerleader of your organisation and team.
  • Present a convincing narrative and a compelling vision about the organisation.
✓ Instil a sense of togetherness, hope, pride and ownership.

....

✓ People like stories: They inform, they involve and they inspire.

....

✓ Embody your philosophy.
✓ Emotionalise your vision.
✓ Show your passion.

....

✓ Balance an atmosphere of negativity with an attitude of positivity: Communicate in a realistic but optimistic manner.

....

✓ Social media for Chief Executives

- Check your employer's policy and profession's guidance.
- Check your personal profile and privacy settings.

✓ Social media literacy is a strong competitive advantage. Use the power of social media for your purpose: networking, knowledge sharing, influencing. Keep in close contact with your communications team.

✓ Listen to patients and staff, engage with people and organisations, communicate your vision and values on social media.

✓ Use social media for video summaries instead of dull reports.

✓ Bear in mind that your social media posts may have an impact on your reputation, career and job because they give access to your experiences, thoughts and opinions.

✓ You have invested brain and time, heart and soul to achieve your goals. But you will nevertheless be disgraced, shamed and humiliated when something goes wrong. And something will most certainly go wrong. In that case, do not be downhearted.

✓ Remain determined.
✓ Remain measured.
✓ Keep going.
✓ Carry on.

✓ Build strong resilience.
✓ Do not panic.
✓ Always stay calm.
✓ Do not take the weight of the world on your shoulders.
✓ Keep your body fit.
✓ Keep your mood up.
✓ Keep your mind sharp.

✓ Recharge your batteries, regularly and routinely.

✓ Practise something arduous, solitary and spartan. Do something other people are not willing to do. Thereby develop willpower, self-elitism and toughness. All great leaders remember times of apparently unrewarded toil.

✓ In your role as Chief Executive, possible threats to your wellbeing include isolation, loneliness, sadness and depression.
  • So take action.
    ▪ Do not make too many personal sacrifices for your job.
    ▪ You need your family and friends, your hobbies and holidays.

✓ Banish solitude.
✓ Do not isolate yourself in an ivory tower.
✓ Reach out.

✓ Do not let your mood dictate your life.
✓ Understand and manage your emotions and your mind.

✓ Do not take things personally. In particular, this includes rejection.

✓ Take criticism, but do not allow others to bury you up to your neck.

✓ React against individuals who blame you for things you cannot change.

✓ Do not take yourself too seriously. Keep a sense of humour. This is a sign of confidence.

✓ You think you have an impossible job, intractable problems and daunting conditions? Face it. Prove otherwise. You know you have a rewarding job, challenging problems and exciting conditions!

✓ The permanent burden of regulators, politicians, the public and media can cause a toxic environment for everyone. Relatively new approaches, including collective leadership, a fearless culture and team responsibility, can create a supportive environment.

✓ As a Chief Executive you can only move mountains when your task is manageable and your tenure is sustainable.
  • Health systems need to overcome the killers of an innovation culture: overcomplex structures, risk aversion, unnecessary hierarchical levels and rapid executive turnover.

✓ Success requires continuity, predictability and consistency of leadership: Organisations rated as outstanding all have a stable leadership structure.

✓ It is an immense privilege to serve the public.
✓ Announce your departure early to allow the board sufficient time to find a suitable replacement.
  • If a Chief Executive steps down too early, he/she is disappointed.
  • If a Chief Executive steps down too late, everybody else is disappointed.
    ▪ If you are stepping down for any reason, do so amid widespread respect and praise.
✓ Make sure there is a smooth handover of responsibilities.

✓ Building takes much longer than destroying: Moving up takes time, going down does not.

✓ You could be shown the revolving door with little warning.
✓ Always remember: Everyone can fail in this environment.
✓ And also: Everyone can make you fail in this environment.

✓ Also remember that many important factors are beyond your control, e.g. a financial crisis. You can be held to account for your own failure, but not for societal failure.

✓ Hope for the best, but plan for the worst.

....

✓ Always (really, always!) have a Plan B (and C!) that you can slip right into if everything goes wrong.

....

✓ Do not look back in anger.
✓ Do not look forward in fear.

....

✓ Live without regrets.

49.5. MEDICAL DIRECTOR

49.5.1. ROLE

ROLE

The role of Medical Director is now more important than ever for a hospital.

....

- Patient safety
- Care quality
- Clinical standards
- Medical leadership
- Medical workforce
- Corporate responsibilities

49.5.2. QUALIFICATION

CAPABILITIES AND QUALITIES

- Intellectual flexibility, broad scanning, political astuteness
- Improving safety, improving quality, improving performance
- Leading change, reconfiguring services, shaping future
- Engaging staff, managing supportively, accepting responsibility
- Working collaboratively, empowering people, building trust
- Communicating effectively, setting objectives, influencing strategies
- Personal integrity, intellectual integrity, professional integrity
- Self belief, self awareness, self management

KEY SKILL AREAS

- Leading professionally
- Planning strategically
- Developing a learning culture
- Developing an improvement methodology
- Influencing wisely
- Operating effectively

STRONG LEARNING CULTURE

- Building a learning workforce
- Embracing an ethic of learning
- Supporting the capacity for learning
- Developing a learning organisation

STRONG IMPROVEMENT METHODOLOGY

▶ Focusing medical vision and clinical strategy on patient safety and care quality
- Aligning values
- Aligning norms
- Aligning attitudes
- Aligning behaviours
- Aligning objectives
- Aligning directions

▶ Focusing organisational goals and improvement activities around medical priorities and national targets

KEY SUCCESS FACTORS

▶ Focusing on patient safety and care quality

▶ Responding flexibly to patients' needs in different settings

▶ Dealing effectively with the volatility, uncertainty, complexity and ambiguity of contemporary healthcare leadership and management

▶ Responding adaptively to rising demand and increasing costs

▶ Improving the organisation's productivity and financial performance

JOB DESCRIPTION

▶ Job title

▶ Site base

▶ Context to appointment
- Background and strategy
- Structure and leadership
- Finance and operations

▶ Role description
- Professional accountability
- Key working relationships
- Role summary

▶ Candidate specification
- Essential requirements
- Desirable attributes

- ▶ Duties and responsibilities
  - Corporate management
  - Medical leadership
  - Clinical and quality governance
  - Medical appraisal and revalidation
  - Clinical work
  - Clinical information
  - Infection prevention and control
  - Research and clinical development
  - Medical education
  - External links
- ▶ Recruitment process
- ▶ Expected timetable

ADDITIONAL INFORMATION

- ▶ Code of conduct
- ▶ Equality and diversity monitoring
- ▶ Fit and proper person requirements
- ▶ Confidentiality and data security
- ▶ Organisation's safeguarding policy

PERSON SPECIFICATION

- ▶ Education, qualifications and training
- ▶ Occupational experience
- ▶ Skills, abilities and knowledge
- ▶ Personal qualities
  - Essential attributes
  - Desirable attributes

SAMPLE PROFILE

- ▶ Professor AB was appointed as Medical Director at CD Hospital Trust in [month/year]. He/she has worked for the NHS as Consultant … at the CD Hospital since [year]. He/she undertook clinical studies at the EF Hospital ([year-year]), the GH Hospital ([year-year]) and the IJ Hospital ([year-year]). He/she gained Fellowship of the Royal College of … in [year]. He/she is a professor at the University of KL. Professor AB's clinical profile is as a … . He/she has an interest in … . He/she has co-authored over … peer reviewed papers, review articles and book chapters, … conference abstracts, … invited lectures, and won several awards in national and international competitions. As Medical Director at CD he/she has responsibility for clinical governance and oversight of the clinical strategy. He/she is a Board Member and Responsible Officer. In [month/year] he/she was awarded the … by the … .

PROFESSIONAL SUPPORT

- ▶ Coaching
- ▶ Mentoring
- ▶ Benchmarking workshop
- ▶ Budgeting workshop
- ▶ Contingency planning
- ▶ Discussions with the Chief Executive
- ▶ Scenario planning
- ▶ Stakeholder planning
- ▶ Team briefings
- ▶ Networks
- ▶ Simulations

STAFF SUPPORT

- ▶ Personal Assistant
- ▶ Deputy Medical Directors
- ▶ Associate Medical Directors
- ▶ Administrative support

OTHER ESSENTIALS

- ▶ Annual salary
- ▶ Medical insurance
- ▶ Malpractice insurance
- ▶ Continuing professional development

- ▶ Academic time off
- ▶ Time for teaching
- ▶ Funds for research
- ▶ Holiday entitlement
- ▶ Disability insurance
- ▶ Retirement benefits

49.5.3. RESPONSIBILITIES

KEY RESULT AREAS

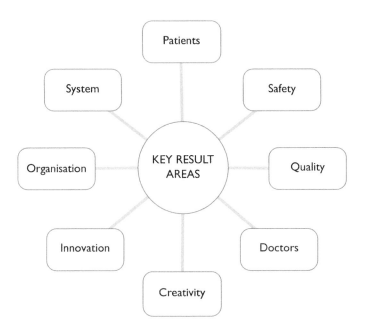

OTHER MAJOR RESPONSIBILITIES

- ▶ Clinical governance
- ▶ Risk management
- ▶ Clinical audit
- ▶ Outcome measurement
- ▶ Academic programmes

▶ Corporate targets

▶ Organisational responsibilities

▶ Annualised job planning schemes

▶ Clinical services strategy

▶ Business planning

▶ Cost improvement initiatives

▶ Mentoring and coaching programmes

COMPLEX ORGANISATIONAL COMMITMENT

▶ System level
  - External stakeholders
  - Regional networks
  - National programmes
▶ Board level
  - Strategic decisions
  - Governance decisions
  - Quality decisions
  - Productivity decisions
  - Operational decisions
▶ Team level
  - Leading teams
  - Transforming services
▶ Individual level
  - Supporting patients
  - Mentoring doctors
  - Managing performance

ENSURING CORPORATE PERFORMANCE

▶ Integral to achieving a vision of excellence
  - Developmental priorities
  - Operational priorities

DEVELOPMENTAL PRIORITIES

▶ Board Assurance Framework
- Based on an integrated governance approach
- Driven by the annual developmental objectives
  ▪ Identifying, controlling and mitigating risks

OPERATIONAL PRIORITIES

▶ Everyday operational priorities
- Business as usual
- Key performance metrics
  ▪ Identifying, controlling and mitigating risks

RESPONSIBILITY AND ACCOUNTABILITY

▶ Important GMC guidance
- 'A guide for doctors reported to the GMC'
- 'A guide for health professionals on how to report a doctor to the GMC'
- 'Confidentiality – Good practice in handling patient information'
- 'Consent – Patients and doctors making decisions together'
- 'Continuing professional development – Guidance for all doctors'
- 'Delegation and referral'
- 'Effective governance to support medical revalidation – A handbook for boards and governing bodies'
- 'Generic professional capabilities framework'
- 'Good medical practice'
- 'Good medical practice framework for appraisal and revalidation'
- 'Guidance for doctors acting as responsible consultants or clinicians'
- 'Guidance on supporting information for appraisal and revalidation'
- 'Guidance to doctors working under system pressure'
- 'How to complain about a doctor'
- 'Leadership and management for all doctors'
- 'Openness and honesty when things go wrong – The professional duty of candour'
- 'Raising and acting on concerns about patient safety'

- 'The GMC protocol for making revalidation recommendations'
- 'The reflective practitioner – Guidance for doctors and medical students'
- 'Writing references'

▶ Doctors are accountable to the GMC for their own conduct and any medical advice they give.
- This includes while they serve as a board member of a decision making body for a health organisation.

▶ The care, dignity and safety of patients must always be the first concern of all doctors, whether or not they have a leadership and management role.

RESPONSIBLE OFFICER'S ROLE

▶ If a doctor is a Responsible Officer within a designated body, he/she has extra responsibilities as set out in the relevant regulations and must take account of any guidance produced by the Department of Health, the General Medical Council or other relevant organisations.

▶ Important Department of Health guidance
- 'The role of the responsible officer'

▶ All doctors should confirm that their indemnity organisation covers the full scope of their practice.
▶ Some roles, such as that of the Responsible Officer, are not covered by all professional indemnity organisations.
▶ Medical Directors should therefore ensure that other indemnity arrangements are in place in this situation.

RESPONSIBLE CONSULTANT'S ROLE

▶ Ensuring that a patient's entire stay in hospital is coordinated

▶ Ensuring that every patient knows who has overall responsibility for their care

▶ Ensuring that responsibility is transferred to another consultant when appropriate

APPRAISAL AND REVALIDATION

▶ Medical Directors participate in an annual appraisal with NHS England leading to revalidation.

▶ Important FMLM guidance
  • 'Supporting information for appraisal and revalidation – Speciality guidance for the leadership and management aspects of a doctor's scope of practice'

▶ If the appraisal process includes academic clinical staff, it should follow the Follett principles
  • 'A review of appraisal, disciplinary and reporting arrangements for senior NHS and university staff with academic and clinical duties'

▶ The patient experience should be at the heart of the annual appraisal, i.e. how patients perceive the quality of the doctor's work.

MENTORING DOCTORS

▶ Principle
  • Mentee guided by the mentor
▶ Method
  • Listening and talking in confidence
▶ Techniques
  • Advising, counselling, encouraging, supporting, teaching

▶ Benefits to the mentee
  • Personal empowerment
  • Personal functionality
  • Personal growth
▶ Benefits to the mentor
  • Sharing of experiences

- Learning with juniors
- Sense of fulfilment
► Benefits to the organisation
  - Job attachment
  - Job performance
  - Job satisfaction

► Mentoring should be available to all doctors.
► Doctors should be mentored in any new role.
► Participation in mentoring should always be voluntary.

WRITING REFERENCES

► If doctors have been asked to or have agreed to write a reference for a colleague, they must follow the GMC guidance in 'Writing references'.

► References must be honest and objective.
► References must include information about competence, performance and conduct.
► References must be accurate and reliable.

► Structure of a reference
  - Introduction
  - Referee
    ▪ Background of referee
    ▪ Relationship to applicant
    ▪ Purpose of reference
  - Skills
    ▪ Academic skills
    ▪ Analytical skills
    ▪ Professional skills
    ▪ Innovation skills
    ▪ Communication skills
    ▪ Presentation skills
    ▪ Interpersonal skills

- Teamwork skills
- Multicultural skills
- International skills
- Management skills
- Leadership skills
- Traits
  - Dedication
  - Initiative
  - Creativity
  - Adaptability
  - Versatility
  - Judgement
  - Decisiveness
  - Persuasiveness
  - Assertiveness
  - Integrity
  - Ethics
  - Character
- Weaknesses
- Goals
- Potential
- Conclusion

▶ Facts must be correct.
▶ Praise must be convincing.
▶ Enthusiasm must be credible.
▶ Evidence must be specific.

49.5.4. TIPS

TIPS FOR MEDICAL DIRECTORS

✓ As a clinician you can help some of the healthcare organisation's patients.
✓ As a Medical Director you can help all of the healthcare organisation's patients.
✓ It is extremely rewarding to be Medical Director of a healthcare organisation.

✓ Active medical involvement in organisational management has a highly positive effect on service quality.

✓ You should thus be a capable, authoritative and visible leadership force in your organisation.

✓ There is no medical-management divide because the intention of medical clinicians and Medical Directors is the same: the best possible patient care.

✓ There are many pathways to becoming a Medical Director.

✓ Few medical leaders are born.

✓ Most medical leaders are made.
   • However, a 'natural inclination' is a huge advantage.

✓ You learn on the job.

✓ You grow with your experience.

✓ Forge sustainable relationships with your executive body.

✓ Stay particularly close to your Chief Executive.

✓ Do not allow other executives to strike deals with medical staff behind your back.

✓ Medical Directors need high credibility and a strong voice within the consultant body.

✓ Demonstrate very strong collegial values.
   • A disconnect between a Medical Director and the consultant body is harmful for the organisation.

✓ Strive to be fair, objective, evidence based, logical and consistent.

✓ Walk the wards and listen.

✓ Listen to your colleagues' concerns and ask for your colleagues' input.

- Leverage teamwork in your organisation.
  - Clinician-to-clinician communication is most powerful.
- Engage colleagues and effect change.

✓ Set an example of professional and compassionate leadership for doctors.

✓ It is vital that you have excellent front line relationships.
✓ Listen very carefully to the experts on the front line.

✓ Be in touch with doctors.
✓ Be in touch with nurses.
  - Conversations with the front line carry weight at board level.
✓ Be accessible.
✓ Be approachable.

✓ Harness the extraordinary leadership potential of front line doctors and nurses.

✓ Bring the front line of healthcare service into the board meetings: Medical engagement correlates with clinical performance.

✓ Maintain clinical practice.

✓ Be willing to help out without being asked.

✓ Your patients are your greatest source of learning.

✓ Being patient-driven is about building a deep understanding of what patients want and what patients need.

✓ Dedicated Medical Directors are powerful patient advocates.

✓ Work towards patients receiving the right care the first time, every time.

....

✓ Help cultivate a loyal patient base.

✓ Make your patients love your hospital.

....

✓ Focus emphatically on patient safety and care quality.
  ● Measure it, promote it, improve it, monitor it – and manage it proactively.

✓ Never compromise on patient safety and care quality.

....

✓ Optimise patient safety without adding complexity, wherever possible.

....

✓ Be a role model for a safety and quality culture.
  ● Focus on medical ethos.
  ● Focus on strong values.
  ● Focus on professional behaviours.
  ● Focus on continuous learning.
  ● Focus on mentoring systems.
  ● Focus on appraisal output.
  ● Focus on standardised processes.
  ● Focus on high reliability.
  ● Focus on measured outcomes.
  ● Focus on team accountability.

....

✓ Zero tolerance for breaches of safety!
  ● If minor breaches are accepted, major failures will follow.

✓ Absolute emphasis on protection from harm!

....

✓ Whenever possible, promote healthcare which is
  ● Free from harm
    ▪ Free from risks
    ▪ Free from side effects
    ▪ Free from downsides
  ● Supported by evidence

- Consistent with values
- Truly necessary
- Not duplicative
- Cost effective

✓ Listen, consider and act on concerns.

✓ Never disregard or dismiss early warnings or signs of safety risks.
✓ Never marginalise or victimise clinical staff or others for raising concerns.

✓ Remember: You could be removed from the medical register for misconduct in a managerial capacity if you put patients at risk.

✓ Health systems need collaborative and transformational leaders as Medical Directors.
- Move away from competition towards collaboration.
- Move away from preservation towards transformation.

✓ Work across professional, functional, sectoral, organisational and geographical boundaries to improve patient care.

✓ Work towards integrated care: Disorganised and disjointed care is wasteful and harmful care – and it is a source of frustration for patients and staff.

✓ Focus on prudent healthcare and realistic medicine.

✓ Look both outside-in and inside-out: You can only lead with a 360 degree view of your organisation.

✓ Look at the whole organisation.
✓ Drive cohesiveness across all sites.
✓ Create a community spirit.

✓ Act in a corporate manner.
✓ Commit to a transparency culture.

✓ Engage multiple stakeholders behind the common purpose.

✓ Medical Directors are catalysts for change.
✓ Lead in innovation, improvement and implementation.
  • Improvement skills are a vehicle for culture change within organisations.
✓ Medical Directors can change the game.

✓ Excel in strategy as well as in execution.
✓ Excel in inspiration as well as in operation.

✓ Expand your vision, every time and everywhere.

✓ Have a truly global perspective.
✓ Look at world class examples.

✓ Remember: True leaders have their eyes on the hill, while others have their eyes on the valley.

✓ Navigate your hospital beyond the line of sight.
✓ Anticipate the invisible.
✓ Think several moves ahead and beyond the horizon.
✓ Expect the unexpected.

✓ Develop a forward-thinking approach to leadership.

✓ Maintain control during unexpected events.
✓ Manage the unexpected with confidence.

✓ Know the headwinds and the tailwinds of your vision.

....

✓ Identify opportunities and alternatives through alertness and agility.
- Have an idea.
- Explore the options.
- Embrace ambiguity.
- Challenge the status quo.
- Strive for new heights.
- Create visions.
- Value the offbeat.
- Focus on innovation.

....

✓ Realistic thinking is the catalyst for positive change.
- Realistic thinking provides a target.
- Realistic thinking provides a plan.
- Realistic thinking gives you credibility.
- Realistic thinking gives you security.
- Realistic thinking reduces the uncertainty.
- Realistic thinking reduces the error.

....

✓ Engage, get involved, join – there are many opportunities.
- Care Quality Commission specialist adviser
- Getting It Right First Time
- Royal Colleges
- Clinical Senates
  - Clinical Senate Council
  - Clinical Senate Forum
- Healthcare charities
- Specialised services clinical reference groups
- Seven day services programme lead

....

✓ When you take the helm you will often need to sail against the wind.

....

✓ Do not expect – or try – to be liked by everybody. Aim for respect instead.

✓ Stop the worry – or fear – that you will not succeed. Act with confidence instead.

....

✓ You cannot – and will not – make everybody happy.

....

✓ Set your personal boundaries and red lines. Make them clear and make them firm.

....

✓ You will need to mediate and negotiate between different interest groups.
   • Exemplary personal standards of conduct and behaviour and excellent communication skills are absolutely essential to achieving the optimum result.

....

✓ Handling difficult doctors requires firmness, Human Resources support, attention to detail and fairness. You should still be caring even if you have to dismiss a doctor.

....

✓ Have a 'learning by doing' approach, a 'yes I can' attitude and a 'just do it' mentality.

....

✓ Opportunities arise every day. Make a substantial contribution. Take initiative, elaborate an idea and make it happen. You ought to be a thinker and a doer.

....

✓ Communication is an act of leadership. Leadership communication must be compelling communication.

....

✓ Adjust your style.

✓ Make sure people understand you.

✓ Speak their language.

....

✓ Read minds, not reports.

✓ Understand needs, not statistics.

....

✓ Address communication shortcomings and improve communication practices. Communicate. Communicate. Communicate. Explain. Explain. Explain. Use the power of talking to people.

✓ You and your hospital can only rise from good to great with disciplined leadership, disciplined staff, disciplined thought and disciplined action.

✓ But: Do not let the aspiration for perfection hinder the need for pragmatism.

✓ Outstanding Medical Directors are role models with the highest performance levels.
  • They exceed expectations in all relevant qualities.
  • They are a true organisational asset.
  • They demonstrate mastery of their current assignment.

✓ And: Outstanding Medical Directors have a lot of red letter days – brimming over with enthusiasm, excitement and exhilaration.

50 HEALTHCARE EXCELLENCE

CHAPTER OVERVIEW

▶ **HEALTHCARE EXCELLENCE**
▶ **OUTSTANDING LEADERS**

HEALTHCARE EXCELLENCE

▶ This chapter is dedicated solely to outstanding leaders: It is they who, at all levels and at all times, create a culture of excellence in healthcare.

OUTSTANDING LEADERS

▶ Outstanding leaders are the cream of the crop.
▶ Outstanding leaders have shifted from success to significance.

▶ Outstanding leaders think and act in a systemic and holistic way.
▶ Outstanding leaders are people centred and relationship oriented.
▶ Outstanding leaders think and act in terms of outcomes and consequences.

▶ Outstanding leaders focus more on people than on objectives.
▶ Outstanding leaders focus more on people's attitudes and engagement than on people's skills and tasks.
▶ Outstanding leaders focus more on team equality and spirit than on team size and background.
▶ Outstanding leaders focus more on challenge than on coaching.

▶ Outstanding leaders delegate autonomy and not just tasks.

▶ Outstanding leaders want the people and the team to carry responsibility.

▶ Outstanding leaders understand people and not just work.

▶ Outstanding leaders serve.

▶ Outstanding leaders are self confident.

▶ Outstanding leaders are extremely focused.

▶ Outstanding leaders enable.

▶ Outstanding leaders convey a high sense of purpose.

▶ Outstanding leaders think and act long term.

▶ Outstanding leaders bring a special meaning to life.

▶ Outstanding leaders put flexibility first.

▶ Outstanding leaders focus on the spirit of law rather than the letter of law.

▶ Outstanding leaders focus on the power of trust rather than the power of control.

▶ Outstanding leaders give people freedom.

▶ Outstanding leaders strive to be role models for other people.

▶ Outstanding leaders put collective needs before their own needs.

▶ Outstanding leaders are in the key position for sustainable success.

▶ Outstanding leaders understand the human psyche – at individual and at group level.

▶ Outstanding leaders excel in personal judgement, intelligence, instinct and gut feeling.

▶ Outstanding leaders know the resulting consequences – at strategic and at operational level.

▶ Outstanding leaders understand what life is all about.

  • Their values, behaviours and goals are deeply rooted, very strong and highly ethical and they extend from the past, through the present and into the future.

▶ Outstanding leaders attain and sustain peak performance levels.

▶ Outstanding leaders have great inner fortitude and awareness.

▶ Outstanding leaders leave a legacy beyond their time.

UNITED KINGDOM

CHAPTER OVERVIEW

- INNOVATION HUB
- APPARENT AFFLUENCE
► MEDICINE
  - UK: HEALTHCARE EXCELLENCE
  - UK: IMPROVING LIVES
  - LONDON: MEDICAL ACHIEVEMENTS
  - CAMBRIDGE: MEDICAL ACHIEVEMENTS
  - OXFORD: MEDICAL ACHIEVEMENTS
  - OTHERS: MEDICAL ACHIEVEMENTS
  - UK: RADIOLOGICAL ACHIEVEMENTS
► PHILOSOPHY
  - GREAT BRITISH PHILOSOPHY
► LITERATURE
  - GREAT BRITISH LITERATURE
► ART
  - GREAT BRITISH ART
► MUSIC
  - GREAT BRITISH MUSIC
  - QUINTESSENTIALLY BRITISH COMPOSITIONS
► SPORT
  - GREAT BRITISH SPORTS
► MEDIA
  - MEDIA
► FARE
  - GREAT BRITISH FOOD
  - GREAT BRITISH DRINKS
► ATTRACTIONS
  - TOURISM
  - LONDON: BOOMING MEGACITY
  - LONDON: TOP ATTRACTIONS
  - LONDON: TOP MUSEUMS
  - LONDON: TOP GALLERIES
  - LONDON: TOP PARKS
  - LONDON: TOP VIEWS
  - LONDON: TOP SHOPPING
  - LONDON: TOP SHOPS

- NORTHERN ENGLAND: TOP ATTRACTIONS
- CENTRAL ENGLAND: TOP ATTRACTIONS
- SOUTHWEST ENGLAND: TOP ATTRACTIONS
- SOUTHEAST ENGLAND: TOP ATTRACTIONS
- ENGLAND: TOP CASTLES AND STATELY HOMES
- EDINBURGH: TOP ATTRACTIONS
- SCOTLAND: TOP ATTRACTIONS
- CARDIFF: TOP ATTRACTIONS
- WALES: TOP ATTRACTIONS
- BELFAST: TOP ATTRACTIONS
- NORTHERN IRELAND: TOP ATTRACTIONS
▶ BRITONS
  - GREAT BRITONS
▶ BRITISH
  - GREAT BRITISH ATTITUDES AND MANNERS
  - GREAT BRITISH SYMBOLS AND INSTITUTIONS
  - GREAT BRITISH PROVERBS AND IDIOMS

OVERVIEW

UNITED KINGDOM

▶ 66 million people
▶ 4 constituent countries

CONSTITUENT COUNTRIES

▶ England
  - Patron saint: St George
  - National capital: London
  - National motto: God and my right
  - National anthem: 'God Save the Queen/King'
    - National anthem of the United Kingdom
  - National flower: Rose

- National tree: Oak
- National animal: Lion
► Scotland
  - Patron saint: St Andrew
  - National capital: Edinburgh
  - National motto: In defence
  - National anthem: 'Flower of Scotland'
  - National flower: Thistle
  - National tree: Scots pine
  - National animal: Unicorn
► Wales
  - Patron saint: St David
  - National capital: Cardiff
  - National motto: Wales forever
  - National anthem: 'Land of My Fathers'
  - National flower: Daffodil
  - National tree: Sessile oak
  - National animal: Red dragon
► Northern Ireland
  - Patron saint: St Patrick
  - National capital: Belfast
  - National motto: Who will separate us?
  - National anthem: 'Londonderry Air'
  - National flower: Shamrock
  - National tree: None
  - National animal: None

UNION FLAG

► The cross of St George, patron saint of England
  - Red cross on a white ground
► The cross of St Andrew, patron saint of Scotland
  - Diagonal white cross on a blue ground
► The cross of St Patrick, patron saint of Ireland
  - Diagonal red cross on a white ground

NATIONAL ANTHEM

God save our gracious Queen/King!
Long live our noble Queen/King!
God save the Queen/King!
Send her/him victorious,
Happy and glorious,
Long to reign over us,
God save the Queen/King!

CORE VALUES

▶ Democracy
▶ Fairness
▶ Freedom
  • Freedom of opinion
  • Freedom of speech
▶ Justice
▶ Law
▶ Liberty
▶ Loyalty
▶ Monarchy
▶ Pragmatism
▶ Property
▶ Responsibility
▶ Tolerance

IMPORTANT DATES

▶ 1 January – New Year's Day
▶ 14 February – Valentine's Day
▶ 1 March – St David's Day
▶ 17 March – St Patrick's Day

- 1 April – April Fool's Day
- 23 April – St George's Day
- 31 October – Halloween
- 5 November – Bonfire Night
- 11 November – Remembrance Day
- 30 November – St Andrew's Day
- 24 December – Christmas Eve
- 25 December – Christmas Day
- 26 December – Boxing Day
- 31 December – New Year's Eve

UK STATISTICS

- Office for National Statistics
  - https://www.ons.gov.uk

HISTORY

OVERVIEW

- Britain was the world's foremost power during the 19th and the early 20th centuries.
- Britain has given the world the most widely spoken language.
- Britain is 'the mother of parliaments'.
- Britain is 'the mother of democracies'.
- Britain formed the Commonwealth of Nations.
- Britain was on the winning side in two world wars.
- Britain twice saved the world from tyranny.
- Britain was the world's first industrialised country.
- Britain had the largest empire in history.
- Britain has not been successfully invaded since the Norman Conquest.
- Britain has invaded almost ninety per cent of the world's countries during its history.

HISTORY

Until AD 43	**Prehistoric Britain**
5000 BC	*Rising sea levels cut Britain off from Europe*
4000 BC	*Farmers settle in Britain*
3100 BC	*Stonehenge* • One of the most ancient and mysterious legacies of Neolithic Britain
2600 BC	*Avebury Stone Circle*
500 BC	*Celts arrive in Britain*
55 BC	*Caesar unsuccessfully invades Britain*
AD 43	**Roman Britain**
AD 43	*Roman Conquest* • Claudius successfully invades Britain
50	*London is founded*
122	*Construction of Hadrian's Wall*
3rd-4th centuries	*Christians appear in Britain* • Constantine is the first Roman emperor to have been converted to Christianity • Constantine's rule is the Golden Age of Roman power in Britain
410	*Romans leave Britain* • End of Roman rule in Britain
430	**Anglo-Saxon Britain**
430-550	*Angles, Saxons and Jutes arrive in Britain*
597	*Augustine becomes the first Archbishop of Canterbury* • The Archbishop of Canterbury is today the principal leader of the Church of England and the symbolic head of the worldwide Anglican Communion
600	*Anglo-Saxon kingdoms are established in Britain* • Anglo-Saxon Heptarchy: East Anglia, Essex, Kent, Mercia, Northumbria, Sussex, Wessex
664	*Synod of Whitby* • Christianity in Britain is allied to Rome
793-1066	*Vikings raid and invade Britain* • The story of the Vikings in Britain is one of conquest, expulsion and reconquest
843	*Kenneth MacAlpin unites the Scots and Picts under his rule*
871	**House of Wessex**

871	*Alfred the Great* • King of Wessex • Alfred successfully defends his kingdom against the Vikings • The Anglo-Saxon kingdoms in England unite under Alfred o The Golden Age of Anglo-Saxon rule • Ruler of England
1066	**Norman Britain**
1066	**House of Normandy**
1066	*William the Conqueror* • Battle of Hastings o William I, Duke of Normandy, defeats Harold II, King of England • Westminster Abbey is first used as coronation church • The Bayeux Tapestry commemorates the battle • The Domesday Book gives a picture of the society in England after the Norman Conquest
1154	**Plantagenet Britain**
1154	**House of Anjou**
1171	*Henry invades Ireland*

1215	*The Magna Carta Libertatum is introduced during King John's rule*
	 • The Magna Carta Libertatum protects the rights of the nobility and restricts the rights of the monarch to collect taxes and to make laws
	 • It is a symbol of freedom, a statement of the liberties of the individual and a protection against despotism
	 • Gradual development of an English parliament
	   o House of Lords
	      ▪ Nobility
	      ▪ Great landowners
	      ▪ Bishops
	   o House of Commons
	      ▪ Knights (smaller landowners)
	      ▪ Wealthy (from towns)
	 • Gradual development of the legal system
	   o The judges are independent of the government
	   o Common law develops by a process of precedence and tradition

1216	**House of Plantagenet**

1284	*England annexes Wales*
	• Statute of Rhuddlan
1314	*Battle of Bannockburn*
	• The Scottish, led by Robert the Bruce, defeat the English
1348	*Black Death*
	• One third of the British population dies
1381	*Peasants' Revolt*
	• The Peasants' Revolt is suppressed and the rebel leaders are executed
1399	**House of Lancaster**
By 1400	*English becomes the preferred language of the royal court and the parliament*
	• Norman-French (spoken by noblemen) and Anglo-Saxon (spoken by peasants) combine to become one English language
1415	*Battle of Agincourt*
	• The English defeat the French in the most famous battle of the Hundred Years War
1453	*The English leave France*
1455	*The Wars of the Roses start between the House of Lancaster and the House of York*
	• House of Lancaster: Red rose
	• House of York: White rose
	• House of Tudor: Red and white rose
1461	**House of York**
1476	*William Caxton introduces the printing press*
1485	**<u>Tudor Britain</u>**
1485	**House of Tudor**
1485	*The Wars of the Roses end between the House of Lancaster and the House of York*
	• Battle of Bosworth Field
	• King Richard III of the House of York is killed
	• Henry Tudor of the House of Lancaster becomes Henry VII
1509	*Henry VIII becomes king*
	• Henry VIII breaks away from the Church of Rome and establishes the Church of England (Anglican Church)
1534	*Acts of Supremacy 1534 and 1559*
	• The Acts of Supremacy establish Henry VIII and subsequent monarchs as the Supreme Head of the Church of England
	o Reformation in England and Wales

1536	*Act of Union between England and Wales*
1553	*Mary I becomes queen*
	• Mary is a devout Catholic, persecutes Protestants and becomes known as Bloody Mary
	• She re-establishes Catholicism in England
1558-1603	*Elizabethan Era*
1558	*Elizabeth I becomes queen*
	• Elizabeth I is the younger daughter of Henry VIII
	• She never marries and becomes known as the Virgin Queen
1560	*Reformation in Scotland*
	• The Church of Scotland (Presbyterian Church) is founded by John Knox
1583	*The University of Edinburgh is established*
1587	*Mary Stuart, Queen of Scots, is executed*
	• Mary is accused of plotting against Elizabeth I
1588	*Elizabeth I defeats the Spanish Armada*
	• England's position as a major trading power and the foremost naval power is secured
	• The Spanish Armada had been sent to conquer England and restore Catholicism
1600	*The East India Company is founded*
1603	**Stuart Britain**
1603	**House of Stuart**
1603	*Union of the Crowns*
	• James I of England, Wales and Ireland and VI of Scotland, Elizabeth's cousin, becomes king
1605	*Gunpowder Plot*
	• The Gunpowder Plot is a failed assassination attempt against James by a group of provincial English Catholics
	• 'Remember, remember, the fifth of November'
	o Guy Fawkes Night
1606	*The Virginia Company is founded*
1609	*Plantation of Ulster*
	• English and Scottish Protestants settle in Ulster, taking over the land from Irish Catholics
1611	*King James Bible*
	• The King James Bible is an English translation of the Christian Bible for the Church of England
1620	*Pilgrim Fathers travel on the Mayflower to the New World*

1628	*Petition of Right* • The Petition of Right contains restrictions on non-parliamentary taxation, the declaration of martial law and imprisonment without cause • It is an important step towards the British system of constitutional monarchy

1642	*English Civil War 1642-1649*
	• Civil war between the Parliamentarian Roundheads, led by Oliver Cromwell, and the Royalist Cavaliers, loyal to Charles I
	  o Battle of Marston Moor 1644
	  o Battle of Naseby 1645

1649-1660	*Interregnum*
1649	*England becomes a republic, called the Commonwealth* • Charles I is executed
1651	*Navigation Act* • The Navigation Act restricts colonial trade to the mother country • It reflects the policy of mercantilism
1653	*Oliver Cromwell becomes Lord Protector*
1660-1688	*Restoration*
1660	*Charles II becomes king* • Restoration of the monarchy
1660	*The Royal Society is formed to promote natural knowledge*
1666	*Great Fire of London*
1670	*The Hudson's Bay Company is founded*
1679	*Habeas Corpus Act* • The Habeas Corpus Act forces the courts to examine the lawfulness of detention in order to safeguard individual liberty and prevent arbitrary imprisonment
1688	*Glorious Revolution* • Influential Protestants ask William of Orange to proclaim himself king
1688	*William of Orange becomes William III of England, Wales and Ireland and II of Scotland*

1689	*Bill of Rights*
	• The Bill of Rights sets out the rights of the parliament and limits the powers of the monarch
	  o Requirement for regular parliaments, freedom of speech and free elections
	• Legislative powers rest with parliament alone
	  o Tories and Whigs are the two main groups in the parliament

1690	*Battle of the Boyne* • William III defeats James II, brother of Charles II, in Ireland • James II flees back to France
1694	*The Bank of England is founded*
1695	*Printing Act* • The end of pre-publication censorship stimulates newspapers
1701	*Act of Settlement* • Under the Act of Settlement, anyone who becomes a Catholic, or who marries one, is disqualified from succeeding to the throne
1707	*Act of Union* • The Act of Union creates Great Britain, the union of England, Wales and Scotland • Scotland keeps its own legal, educational and religious systems
1713	*Treaty of Utrecht* • War of the Spanish Succession 1701-1714 • The Treaty of Utrecht marks the rise of the power of Britain and the Empire at the expense of both France and Spain • Spain cedes Gibraltar and Minorca to Britain
1714	**Georgian Britain**
1714	**House of Hanover**
1721	*Robert Walpole becomes the first British prime minister*

1746	*Battle of Culloden*
	• George II defeats Bonnie Prince Charlie
	• The clans lose much of their power and influence
	   o Chieftains become landlords
	   o Clansmen become tenants

1763	*Treaty of Paris* • Seven Years' War 1756-1763 • The Treaty of Paris marks the beginning of British dominance outside Europe • Britain gains much of France's possessions in North America
1764	*Spinning Jenny* • James Hargreaves

1769	*Steam engine* • James Watt • Industrial Revolution o Textiles o Steel o Coal o Railways o Steamships • The Enlightenment o Everyone should have the right to their own political and religious beliefs • Overseas colonisation
1775	*American War of Independence between the American colonial and the British forces 1775-1783*
1795-1837	*Regency Era*
1800	*Act of Union* • The Act of Union unifies Great Britain and Ireland
1801	*The London Stock Exchange is founded*
1805	*Battle of Trafalgar* • Admiral Horatio Nelson defeats the combined fleets of the French Navy and the Spanish Navy
1807	*Slave Trade Act* • The Slave Trade Act abolishes the slave trade in the British Empire
1815	*Battle of Waterloo* • The Duke of Wellington defeats the French army and Emperor Napoleon
1832	*First Reform Act* • The First Reform Act increases the number of people with the right to vote and abolishes rotten and pocket boroughs
1833	*Slavery Abolition Act* • The Slavery Abolition Act abolishes slavery throughout the British Empire
1834	*The Conservative Party is founded (formerly Tories)*
1836	*The University of London is established*
1837	**Victorian Britain**
1837	*Victoria becomes queen*
1842	*Treaty of Nanking* • First Opium War 1839-1842 • China cedes Hong Kong to Britain

1851	*The Crystal Palace houses the Great Exhibition*
1859	*The Liberal Party is founded (formerly Whigs)*
1867	*Second Reform Act* • The Second Reform Act creates more urban seats in the parliament and reduces the amount of property that people needed to have before they could vote
1868	*The Trades Union Congress is founded*
1876	*Victoria becomes Empress of India*
1884	*Third Reform Act* • The Third Reform Act further extends suffrage
1900	*The Labour Party is founded*

1901	*Victoria dies*
	
	• The British Empire (1815-1914) is the largest empire of all time
	
	  o It covers a quarter of the world's land
	
	  o It covers a fifth of the world's population
	
	• It is said that the sun never sets on the British Empire

1901	**Edwardian Britain**
1901	**House of Saxe-Coburg-Gotha** • **House of Windsor from 1917**
1906	*David Lloyd George introduces the Liberal welfare reforms (1906-1914)*

1911	*Parliament Act*
	
	• The House of Commons establishes its formal dominance over the House of Lords
	
	• The Parliament Act 1911 limits the legislation blocking powers of the House of Lords
	
	  o The Lords are allowed to delay but not to veto bills passed by the Commons
	
	  o The Lords lose the right to question financial legislation passed by the Commons

1914-1918	**World War I**
1918	**Inter-War Britain**
1918	*Representation of the People Act* • The Representation of the People Act is the first to include all men in the political system and begins the inclusion of women
1921	*Anglo-Irish Treaty* • The Anglo-Irish Treaty provides for the establishment of the Irish Free State as a self governing dominion • It gives Northern Ireland the option to opt out of the Irish Free State, which it exercises

417

1922	The British Broadcasting Corporation is founded
1922	Ireland is separated into two countries
1926	Balfour Declaration • The Balfour Declaration declares the United Kingdom and the dominions to be autonomous communities within the British Empire, equal in status, united by a common allegiance to the Crown, and freely associated as members of the British Commonwealth of Nations
1928	Representation of the People (Equal Franchise) Act • The Equal Franchise Act grants equal voting rights to men and women • Men and women have the right to vote at the age of 21
1931	Statute of Westminster • The Statute of Westminster becomes the statutory embodiment of the principles of equality and common allegiance to the Crown as set out in the Balfour Declaration • It is an important step in the development of the dominions as separate states
1934	The Scottish National Party is founded
1939-1945	**World War II**
1940	Winston Churchill becomes prime minister
1940	Battle of Britain • The Royal Air Force wins the crucial aerial battle against the German air force • 'This was their finest hour' (Winston Churchill)
1944	Education Act • The Education Act, also known as 'Butler Act', provides free secondary education
1945	**Post-War Britain**
1945	Clement Attlee becomes prime minister • The welfare state • Nationalisation of industries
1947	Independence is granted to nine colonies of the Empire, including India, Pakistan and Ceylon
1947-1967	Independence is granted to other colonies of the Empire in the Caribbean, Pacific and Africa
1948	Aneurin Bevan spearheads the establishment of the National Health Service
1949	The Irish Free State becomes a republic

1949	Parliament Act
	• The Parliament Act 1949 further limits the power of the Lords by reducing the time that they can delay bills to one year
1951	Winston Churchill returns as prime minister
1952	Elizabeth II becomes queen
1958	Life Peerages Act
	• The prime minister is given the power to nominate life peers
1969	The Troubles begin in Northern Ireland
1969	Representation of the People Act
	• The voting age is reduced to 18 for men and women
1979	Margaret Thatcher becomes prime minister
	• Deregulation
	• Monetarism
	• Privatisation
1998	Good Friday Agreement
	• The Good Friday Agreement is a major political development in the Northern Irish peace process
1998	Devolution Acts
	• Some powers are devolved from central government to give people in Scotland, Wales and Northern Ireland more control over domestic matters

ARCHIVES

▶ National Archives
  • https://www.nationalarchives.gov.uk

POLITICS

POLITICAL SYSTEM

▶ Britain is considered 'the mother of parliaments' and 'the mother of democracies'.

▶ Parliamentary democracy
▶ Constitutional monarchy
▶ Unwritten constitution

▶ Sources of the constitution
- Statutes and Acts
- Case and Common Law
- Royal Prerogative
- Conventions
- Institutional Rules

CONSTITUTIONAL INSTITUTIONS

▶ Monarch
- https://www.royal.uk
- Heads the state
- Advises the government
    - Has the right to encourage
    - Has the right to be consulted
    - Has the right to warn
- Undertakes constitutional and representational duties
- Ensures stability and continuity
- Provides identity and pride

▶ Parliament
- https://www.parliament.uk
- Examines, debates and approves new laws
- Checks the work of government
    - Scrutiny
- Enables the government to raise taxes

▶ Parliament
- House of Commons: Elected lower chamber
    - Members of Parliament
        - Represent their constituency
        - Debate national issues
        - Control the finances
        - Create new laws
        - Scrutinise the government
        - Redress private grievances

- House of Lords: Unelected upper chamber
  - Lords Spiritual, Lords Temporal (Life Peers, Hereditary Peers)
    - Check laws
    - Suggest amendments
    - Propose laws
    - Provide a forum of expertise
    - Challenge the actions of government
    - Have the power of veto

▶ The House of Commons is the sounding board for the nation.

▶ The House of Lords has a deliberative, legislative and constitutional function.
  - It has the power to delay a bill for a period of one year.
  - It has the power of veto over any proposal to extend the maximum duration of Parliament beyond five years.

▶ The House of Commons has the power to overrule the House of Lords.

▶ Speaker
  - Is a Member of Parliament
  - Chairs the House of Commons and is expected to be politically impartial
  - Keeps order during political debates
▶ Lord Speaker
  - Chairs the House of Lords and is expected to be politically impartial

▶ Hansard is the official report of Parliament.

▶ HM Government
  - https://www.gov.uk
  - Runs the country
  - Develops and implements policy
  - Drafts the laws

- ▶ Prime Minister
  - • https://www.gov.uk/government/organisations/prime-ministers-office-10-downing-street
  - • Leads the government
    - ▪ Chief executive
    - ▪ Chief policy-maker
    - ▪ Party-political leader
    - ▪ First citizen
  - • Represents the government
  - • Appoints and dismisses Ministers of the Cabinet
  - • Presides over Cabinet
  - • Advises the Monarch

- ▶ HM Government
  - • Prime Minister
  - • Cabinet
    - ▪ Ministers
  - • Civil servants
- ▶ HM Most Loyal Opposition
  - • Opposition Leader
  - • Shadow Cabinet
    - ▪ Shadow Ministers

- ▶ Cabinet as the collective decision making body of the government

- ▶ Ways of scrutinising government
  - • Committees
  - • Questions
  - • Ombudsman

LEGISLATION PROCESS

- ▶ House of Commons
  - • First reading
  - • Second reading

- Committee stage
- Report stage
- Third reading

▶ House of Lords
  - First reading
  - Second reading
  - Committee stage
  - Report stage
  - Third reading

▶ Monarch
  - Royal Assent

▶ Both Houses must agree on the text of a bill before it can become an Act.

▶ The House of Lords cannot amend money bills.

DEVOLVED ADMINISTRATIONS

▶ Scotland
  - Scottish Parliament at Holyrood, Edinburgh
    - Civil and criminal law
    - Additional tax raising powers
    - Health
    - Education
    - Etc.
  - http://www.gov.scot
▶ Wales
  - National Assembly for Wales in the Senedd, Cardiff
    - Health
    - Education
    - Etc.
  - http://gov.wales
▶ Northern Ireland
  - Northern Ireland Assembly at Stormont, Belfast
    - Health

- Education
- Etc.
- https://www.northernireland.gov.uk

▶ Policy and laws governing foreign affairs, defence, taxation, immigration and social security remain under central UK government control.
▶ The central UK government has the power to suspend all devolved assemblies.

LOCAL GOVERNMENT

▶ County councils
▶ District, borough and city councils
▶ Unitary authorities
▶ Parish, community and town councils

ELECTORAL SYSTEM

▶ General elections
- Held at least every five years
- Majority representation
- System called 'first past the post'
▶ By-elections
- When a Member of Parliament dies or resigns
▶ Devolved elections
- Every five years
▶ Local elections
- Once a year

LAW

LEGAL SYSTEM

▶ History of English Law
- Common Law
- Equity

- ▶ Classification of English Law
  - Private Law
  - Public Law
- ▶ Sources of English Law
  - Case Law and Precedents
  - Legislation and Statute Law
  - Custom
  - Books of Authority

- ▶ Civil Courts
  - Minor cases
    - England, Wales, Northern Ireland: County Court
    - Scotland: Sheriff Court
  - Serious cases
    - England, Wales, Northern Ireland: High Court
    - Scotland: Court of Session

- ▶ Criminal Courts
  - Minor cases
    - England, Wales, Northern Ireland: Magistrates' Court
      - Lay magistrates or district judge
    - Scotland: Justice of the Peace Court
  - Serious cases
    - England, Wales, Northern Ireland: Crown Court
      - Judge and jury
    - Scotland: Sheriff Court
      - Sheriff and jury

- ▶ Superior Courts
  - High Court
  - Court of Appeal
  - Supreme Court

- ▶ The Supreme Court is the highest appellate court in all matters under English, Welsh and Northern Irish law and under Scottish civil law.
  - Points of law of general public importance
- ▶ The High Court of Judiciary is the highest appellate court in all matters under Scottish criminal law.

- ▶ Previously, the highest appellate court was formed by the Lords of Appeal in Ordinary – the 'Law Lords' – appointed by the monarch, usually from the ranks of the senior judiciary.
- ▶ The Constitutional Reform Act provided for the establishment of the Supreme Court to separate the senior judges from Parliament.

- ▶ The Judicial Committee of the Privy Council developed as the highest appellate court for civil and criminal cases from across the British Empire.
- ▶ Today, it still performs this function for many Commonwealth countries, as well as for British overseas territories, the crown dependencies and military sovereign base areas.

ECONOMY

BUSINESS PRINCIPLES

- ▶ Core principles of the political, legal and regulatory framework in the United Kingdom
  - Accountability
  - Flexibility
  - Proportionality
  - Transparency
- ▶ International reputation of the political, legal and regulatory framework in the United Kingdom
  - Certainty
  - Consistency
  - Continuity
  - Stability

INTERNATIONAL GATEWAY

▶ Fifth largest economy in the world currently

▶ Largest economy in Western Europe by 2030

▶ Largest air transport system in Europe

▶ London ranked top in the world for the efficiency, reliability and safety of its transport network

▶ Most improved rail network in Europe

▶ First in Europe for foreign direct investment

▶ First in Europe for online retail business

GLOBAL TRADING

▶ First in Europe for business friendly environment

▶ First of Europe's major economies for overall tax position

▶ First in Europe for investor confidence

▶ First in Europe for holding companies

▶ First in Europe for headquarters

▶ Country of choice for large multinational companies

▶ World leader in professional and business services

- Accountancy
- Law
- Advertising
- Audit

▶ First of Europe's major economies for superfast broadband service

- Cloud computing
- Flexible working
- Wide area network connectivity
- Internet protocol telephony
- Real time information sharing
- Social media
- Online sales

▶ London largest city in Europe

▶ London business capital of Europe

▶ London shopping capital of the world

▶ London leading financial centre of the world

▶ London most international stock exchange in the world

▶ London largest centre for international banking in the world

▶ London largest digital cluster in Europe

TALENT MAGNET

▶ First in Western Europe for adults with tertiary education

▶ First in Europe for number of graduates

▶ First in the world for the quality of its universities

- Four of the top six universities in the world
  - Oxford
  - Cambridge
  - University College London
  - Imperial College London

▶ World leader in life sciences

- First in Europe for life sciences graduates
- Three of the top four medical faculties in the world
- First in the world for pharmaceutical companies' operations

▶ First in Europe for leading MBA institutions

▶ First among the major economies in Europe for global talent

- Human capital as the engine of economic growth
  - Talent
  - Ability to innovate
  - Creativity

▶ Workplace of choice for graduates in Europe

- Brain gain as a result of attracting talent

▶ First in Europe for the creative economy

- Television
- Film
- Fashion
- Advertising sector
- Mobile content
- Video games

▶ First among the major economies for workforce in professional occupations

▶ Only major economy in Europe with a growing labour force

▶ Second among the world's major economies for labour market efficiency

▶ First among the Western European economies for competitive labour costs

▶ First among the major economies in Europe for wage tax
  ● Income tax rate
  ● Social security contributions

▶ London the top magnet for top talent in the world

INNOVATION HUB

▶ Top major economy in the Global Innovation Index

▶ Highest research productivity among the top research nations in terms of publications and citations

▶ Second for Nobel Prizes in scientific disciplines

▶ First in Western Europe for effective cooperation between universities and business

▶ First in the Global Intellectual Property Index

▶ First in the G20 for knowledge intensive jobs

APPARENT AFFLUENCE

▶ Number one destination for the world's super rich
  ● UK more billionaires per head of population than any other country
  ● London more billionaires per head of population than any other city

MEDICINE

UK: HEALTHCARE EXCELLENCE

▶ World leader in life sciences
  ● First in Europe for life sciences graduates
  ● Three of the top four medical faculties in the world
  ● First in the world for pharmaceutical companies' operations

▶ Highest performing health system in a group of the most important industrialised countries
  ● Number one in quality care
    ▪ Effective care
    ▪ Safe care

- Co-ordinated care
    - Patient-centred care
  - Number one in access
  - Number one in efficient care
  - Number one in values
  - Number one in care process
  - Number one in equity

▶ The National Health Service
  - One of the proudest achievements of the country
  - A health system of the people, by the people and for the people
  - A symbol of what is Great about Britain

UK: IMPROVING LIVES

▶ A record of success in
  - Discoveries
  - Inventions
  - Innovations
  - Improvements

LONDON: MEDICAL ACHIEVEMENTS

▶ ACE inhibitors – John Vane
▶ Acetylcholine – Henry Dale
▶ Acquired immunological tolerance, 'father of transplantation' – Peter Medawar
▶ Addison's disease – Thomas Addison
▶ Aldosterone – Sylvia Simpson and James Tait
▶ Anatomical substrates for brain functions – David Ferrier
▶ Bankart lesion – Arthur Bankart
▶ Bence Jones protein – Henry Bence Jones
▶ Beta blockers, important principles of drug treatment – James Black
▶ Breast cancer gene BRCA2 – Michael Stratton
▶ Cataract surgery – Harold Ridley
▶ Circulation – William Harvey

- ▶ Clinical cardiac electrophysiology – Thomas Lewis
- ▶ Cooper's ligaments – Astley Cooper
- ▶ Cowper's gland – William Cowper
- ▶ Echophonocardiography – Aubrey Leatham
- ▶ Effects of smoking on health – Richard Doll and Austin Bradford Hill
- ▶ Endotracheal anaesthesia, anaesthetic equipment – Ivan Magill
- ▶ 'Father of epidemiology' – John Snow
- ▶ 'Father of epileptology' – John Hughlings Jackson
- ▶ 'Father of medical statistics' – Austin Bradford Hill
- ▶ 'Father of metabolic medicine' – Archibald Garrod
- ▶ 'Father of plastic surgery' – Harold Gillies
- ▶ 'Father of tropical medicine' – Patrick Manson
- ▶ Fibre optics – Harold Hopkins and Narinder Kapany
- ▶ First human ECG – Alexander Muirhead
- ▶ First practical ECG – Augustus Waller
- ▶ First serological HIV test – Robin Weiss
- ▶ Gout – Alfred Baring Garrod
- ▶ 'Gray's Anatomy' – Henry Gray
- ▶ H2 receptor antagonists – James Black
- ▶ Heart transplantation – Magdi Yacoub
- ▶ Holography – Dennis Gabor
- ▶ Hormone concept – William Bayliss and Ernest Starling
- ▶ Law of the heart – Ernest Starling
- ▶ Mitral valve surgery – Russell Brock
- ▶ Pacemaker – Aubrey Leatham
- ▶ Penicillin – Alexander Fleming
- ▶ Peristalsis – William Bayliss and Ernest Starling
- ▶ Prostaglandins – John Vane
- ▶ Quantal neurotransmitter release – Bernard Katz
- ▶ Rheumatoid arthritis – Alfred Baring Garrod
- ▶ Secretin – William Bayliss and Ernest Starling
- ▶ Sharpey's fibres – William Sharpey
- ▶ Surgical techniques – Samuel Sharp
- ▶ TNF inhibitors – Marc Feldmann and Ravinder Maini
- ▶ Vitamin D – Edward Mellanby

CAMBRIDGE: MEDICAL ACHIEVEMENTS

▶ Action potential – Alan Hodgkin and Andrew Huxley
▶ ATPase – John Walker
▶ Clinical thermometer – Clifford Allbutt
▶ DNA double helix structure – Francis Crick
▶ Electron crystallography – Aaron Klug
▶ Embryonic stem cells – Martin Evans
▶ Function of neurons – Edgar Adrian
▶ In vitro fertilisation – Robert Edwards and Patrick Steptoe
▶ Monoclonal antibodies – César Milstein
▶ Programmed cell death – John Sulston
▶ Protein sequencing, insulin structure, DNA sequencing – Frederick Sanger
▶ Protein structure – John Kendrew and Max Perutz
▶ Protein X-ray crystallography – Dorothy Hodgkin
▶ Transplantation surgery, cyclosporine trials – Roy Calne
▶ Vitamin concept – Frederick Gowland Hopkins

OXFORD: MEDICAL ACHIEVEMENTS

▶ Antibody structure – Rodney Porter
▶ Function of neurons – Charles Sherrington
▶ Knee replacement – John Goodfellow and John O'Connor
▶ Thalassaemia – David Weatherall

OTHERS: MEDICAL ACHIEVEMENTS

▶ Aberdeen
  • Apoptosis – Andrew Wyllie
  • Endorphins – Hans Kosterlitz
▶ Belfast
  • Portable defibrillator – Frank Pantridge
▶ Birmingham
  • 'Father of gynaecology', technique of salpingectomy – Lawson Tait
  • Vitamin C – Norman Haworth

- ▶ Cardiff
  - Corneal graft – Tudor Thomas
  - Evidence based medicine – Archibald Cochrane
- ▶ Dundee
  - Minimally invasive surgery – Alfred Cuschieri
  - Tumour suppressor p53 – David Lane
- ▶ Edinburgh
  - Chloroform – James Young Simpson
  - First coronary care unit – Desmond Julian
  - Hepatitis B vaccine – Kenneth Murray
- ▶ Glasgow
  - Antiseptic surgery – Joseph Lister
  - Glasgow coma scale – Bryan Jennett and Graham Teasdale
  - Neurological mapping of brain lesions – William Macewen
- ▶ Leicester
  - DNA fingerprinting, DNA profiling – Alec Jeffreys
- ▶ Liverpool
  - Malaria – Ronald Ross
- ▶ Manchester
  - Contraceptive pill – Herchel Smith
  - Hip replacement – John Charnley
  - Medical ethics – Thomas Percival
- ▶ Sheffield
  - Bisphosphonates – Graham Russell
  - Citric acid cycle – Hans Krebs
- ▶ Southampton
  - Anti IgE asthma therapy – Stephen Holgate

UK: RADIOLOGICAL ACHIEVEMENTS

- ▶ Aberdeen
  - Positron emission tomography – John Mallard
- ▶ Glasgow
  - Ultrasonography – Ian Donald
  - World's first radiology department – John Mcintyre

► London
  - Computed tomography – Godfrey Hounsfield
  - Electromagnetism – Michael Faraday
  - Radiographic standardisation – Kathleen Clark
  - Vacuum tube – William Crookes
  - World's first body CT scanner – Louis Kreel
  - World's first head CT scanner – James Ambrose
  - World's first international radiology congress – Charles Thurston Holland
  - World's first radiology society – Silvanus Thompson
  - World's first scientific radiology journal – Sydney Rowland
  - X-ray crystallography – William Bragg
► Nottingham
  - Magnetic resonance imaging – Peter Mansfield

PHILOSOPHY

GREAT BRITISH PHILOSOPHY

► David Hume – Empiricism
► Francis Bacon – Empiricism
► Jeremy Bentham – Utilitarianism
► John Locke – Liberalism
► John Stuart Mill – Liberalism
► Thomas Hobbes – 'Leviathan'

LITERATURE

GREAT BRITISH LITERATURE

► Agatha Christie – 'And Then There Were None', 'Death on the Nile', 'Murder on the Orient Express', 'The Mousetrap', 'The Murder of Roger Ackroyd'
► Aldous Huxley – 'Brave New World'
► Alfred Tennyson – 'Ulysses'
► Arthur Conan Doyle – Sherlock Holmes
► Benjamin Jonson – 'Bartholomew Fair', 'Every Man in His Humour'

▶ Charles Dickens – 'A Christmas Carol', 'David Copperfield', 'Great Expectations', 'Oliver Twist', 'The Pickwick Papers'

▶ Charlotte Brontë – 'Jane Eyre'

▶ Christopher Marlowe – 'The Tragical History of Doctor Faustus'

▶ Daniel Defoe – 'Robinson Crusoe'

▶ Daphne du Maurier – 'Rebecca', 'The Birds'

▶ David Herbert Lawrence – 'Lady Chatterley's Lover', 'Sons and Lovers'

▶ Dylan Thomas – 'Under Milk Wood'

▶ Edgar Wallace – Crime novels

▶ Edward Morgan Forster – 'A Passage to India', 'A Room with a View'

▶ Emily Brontë – 'Wuthering Heights'

▶ Geoffrey Chaucer – 'The Canterbury Tales'

▶ George Eliot – 'Middlemarch', 'The Mill on the Floss'

▶ George Gordon, Lord Byron – 'She Walks in Beauty'

▶ George Orwell – 'Animal Farm', 'Nineteen Eighty-Four'

▶ Graham Greene – 'Brighton Rock', 'Our Man in Havana', 'The Third Man'

▶ Harold Pinter – 'The Homecoming'

▶ Henry Fielding – 'The History of Tom Jones, a Foundling'

▶ Ian Fleming – James Bond

▶ James Matthew Barrie – 'Peter Pan'

▶ Jane Austen – 'Pride and Prejudice', 'Sense and Sensibility'

▶ Joanne Rowling – Harry Potter

▶ John Boynton Priestley – 'An Inspector Calls'

▶ John Keats – Odes

▶ John le Carré – 'The Spy Who Came in from the Cold'

▶ John Milton – 'Paradise Lost'

▶ John Osborne – 'Look Back in Anger'

▶ John Ronald Reuel Tolkien – 'The Hobbit', 'The Lord of the Rings'

▶ Lewis Carroll – 'Alice's Adventures in Wonderland'

▶ Mary Shelley – 'Frankenstein'

▶ Percy Bysshe Shelley – 'Ode to the West Wind', 'The Cloud', 'To a Skylark'

▶ Robert Burns – 'Auld Lang Syne'

▶ Robert Louis Stevenson – 'Strange Case of Dr Jekyll and Mr Hyde', 'Treasure Island'

▶ Rudyard Kipling – 'The Jungle Book'

▶ Samuel Johnson – 'A Dictionary of the English Language'

435

- ▶ Samuel Taylor Coleridge – 'The Rime of the Ancient Mariner'
- ▶ Thomas Hardy – 'Far from the Madding Crowd'
- ▶ Virginia Woolf – 'A Room of One's Own'
- ▶ Walter Scott – 'Ivanhoe', 'Rob Roy', 'The Heart of Midlothian', 'The Lady of the Lake', 'Waverley'
- ▶ William Blake – 'Jerusalem'
- ▶ William Golding – 'Lord of the Flies'
- ▶ William Makepeace Thackeray – 'Vanity Fair'
- ▶ William Shakespeare – 'A Midsummer Night's Dream', 'As You Like It', 'Hamlet', 'Henry V', 'Julius Caesar', 'King Lear', 'Macbeth', 'Much Ado About Nothing', 'Othello', 'Richard III', 'Romeo and Juliet', Sonnets, 'The Merchant of Venice', 'The Merry Wives of Windsor'
- ▶ William Wordsworth – 'Daffodils', 'The Prelude'

ART

GREAT BRITISH ART

- ▶ Charles Rennie Mackintosh
- ▶ George Frederick Watts
- ▶ George Romney
- ▶ George Stubbs
- ▶ John Constable
- ▶ John Everett Millais
- ▶ Joseph Mallord William Turner
- ▶ Joshua Reynolds
- ▶ Thomas Gainsborough
- ▶ William Hogarth

MUSIC

GREAT BRITISH MUSIC

- ▶ Classical
  - • Benjamin Britten
  - • Edward Elgar

- Gustav Holst
- Henry Purcell
- Hubert Parry
- Ralph Vaughan Williams

▶ Modern
- Adele
- Amy Macdonald
- Amy Winehouse
- Cliff Richard
- Culture Club
- David Bowie
- Depeche Mode
- Dire Straits
- Duran Duran
- Elton John
- Faithless
- Genesis
- New Order
- Oasis
- Pet Shop Boys
- Pink Floyd
- Queen
- Roxy Music
- Spandau Ballet
- Take That
- The Beatles
- The Police
- The Rolling Stones
- The Who
- Wham
- Yes

▶ Musical
- Andrew Lloyd Webber

QUINTESSENTIALLY BRITISH COMPOSITIONS

- ▶ 'Auld Lang Syne'
- ▶ 'Enigma Variations'
- ▶ 'Fantasia on British Sea Songs'
- ▶ 'I Vow to Thee, My Country'
- ▶ 'Jerusalem'
- ▶ 'Land of Hope and Glory'
- ▶ 'Pomp and Circumstance Marches'
- ▶ 'Rule, Britannia!'
- ▶ 'The British Grenadiers'
- ▶ 'The Crown of India Suite'
- ▶ 'The White Cliffs of Dover'

SPORT

GREAT BRITISH SPORTS

- ▶ Badminton
- ▶ Billiards
- ▶ Bowling
- ▶ Cricket
- ▶ Croquet
- ▶ Darts
- ▶ Football
- ▶ Golf
- ▶ Hockey
- ▶ Polo
- ▶ Rowing
- ▶ Rugby
- ▶ Snooker
- ▶ Squash
- ▶ Tennis

MEDIA

MEDIA

▶ Press
- Newspapers
  - ▪ 'Financial Times'
  - ▪ 'The Daily Telegraph'
    - Sunday: 'The Sunday Telegraph'
  - ▪ 'The Guardian'
    - Sunday: 'The Observer'
  - ▪ 'The Times'
    - Sunday: 'The Sunday Times'
- Magazines
  - ▪ 'The Economist'
  - ▪ 'The Spectator'
  - ▪ 'The Week'

▶ Radio
- BBC

▶ Television
- BBC 1
- BBC 2
- ITV
- Channel 4
- Channel 5
- Sky

FARE

GREAT BRITISH FOOD

▶ Afternoon Tea
▶ Apple Crumble
▶ Bacon Butty
▶ Bangers and Mash
▶ Beef Wellington

- ▶ Black Pudding
- ▶ Bread and Butter Pudding
- ▶ Bubble and Squeak
- ▶ Cauliflower Cheese
- ▶ Cheddar Cheese
- ▶ Chicken and Mushroom Pie
- ▶ Chicken Tikka Masala
- ▶ Christmas Plum Pudding with Brandy Butter
- ▶ Christmas Turkey, Chestnut Stuffing and Cranberry Sauce
- ▶ Chutneys
- ▶ Clapshot
- ▶ Clotted Cream
- ▶ Cock-a-Leekie Soup
- ▶ Coddled Eggs
- ▶ Cornish Pasty
- ▶ Cornish Potato Cakes
- ▶ Cream Tea
- ▶ Crisps
- ▶ Crumpets
- ▶ Cullen Skink
- ▶ Cumberland Sausage
- ▶ Custard
- ▶ Double Gloucester Cheese
- ▶ Dumplings
- ▶ Eton Mess
- ▶ Fish and Chips
- ▶ Flapjack
- ▶ Fudge
- ▶ Full Breakfast
- ▶ Gentleman's Relish
- ▶ Haggis
- ▶ Hog's Pudding
- ▶ Hot Cross Buns
- ▶ Jam Roly-Poly
- ▶ Jellied Eels
- ▶ Kedgeree

- ► Kippers
- ► Lancashire Hotpot
- ► Lemon Curd
- ► Lemon Meringue Pie
- ► Lemon Syllabub
- ► Marmite
- ► Mince Pie
- ► Mint Cake
- ► Muffins
- ► Mulligatawny Soup
- ► Mushy Peas
- ► Oysters and Stout
- ► Piccalilli
- ► Pickled Onions
- ► Ploughman's Lunch
- ► Pork Pie
- ► Porridge
- ► Queen of Puddings
- ► Red Leicester Cheese
- ► Rice Pudding
- ► Roast Beef, Yorkshire Pudding and Horseradish Sauce
- ► Roast Lamb, Apricot Stuffing and Mint Sauce
- ► Roast Pork with Crackling, Apple Sauce and Stuffing
- ► Sandwiches
- ► Scones
- ► Scotch Broth
- ► Scotch Eggs
- ► Scouse
- ► Shepherd's Pie
- ► Shortbread
- ► Smoked Haddock
- ► Spiced Baked Apples
- ► Sponge Pudding
- ► Stilton Cheese
- ► Stinking Bishop Cheese
- ► Tartare Sauce

- ▶ Toad-in-the-Hole
- ▶ Toast and Marmalade
- ▶ Treacle Tart
- ▶ Ulster Fry
- ▶ Welsh Cakes
- ▶ Welsh Laverbread
- ▶ Welsh Rarebit
- ▶ Wensleydale Cheese
- ▶ Worcestershire Sauce

GREAT BRITISH DRINKS

- ▶ Ale
- ▶ Cider
- ▶ Gin and Tonic
- ▶ Ginger Beer
- ▶ Pimm's
- ▶ Port Wine
- ▶ Punch
- ▶ Scotch Whisky
- ▶ Tea

ATTRACTIONS

TOURISM

- ▶ VisitBritain
  - • https://www.visitbritain.com
- ▶ London tourism
  - • https://www.visitlondon.com
- ▶ England tourism
  - • https://www.visitengland.com
- ▶ Scotland tourism
  - • https://www.visitscotland.com

- Wales tourism
  - http://www.visitwales.com
- Northern Ireland tourism
  - https://discovernorthernireland.com

LONDON: BOOMING MEGACITY

- Most popular city in the world
- Largest city in Europe
- Business capital of Europe
- Top magnet for top talent in the world
- Leading medical faculties in the world
- Leading financial centre in the world
- Largest centre for international banking in the world
- Shopping capital of the world
- Busiest airport in Europe
- World's largest premium travel market
- Largest digital cluster in Europe

LONDON: TOP ATTRACTIONS

- Barbican
- BBC Broadcasting House
- Big Ben
- Borough Market
- British Library
- Buckingham Palace
  - Changing of the Guard
- Canary Wharf
- Chelsea Physic Garden
- Chinatown
- Churchill War Rooms
- Covent Garden
- Eton College
- Gherkin
- Greenwich
  - Cutty Sark

- ▶ Royal Mews
  - Diamond Jubilee State Coach
- ▶ Royal Opera House
- ▶ Sea Life London Aquarium
- ▶ Shard
- ▶ Somerset House
- ▶ Southbank and Bankside
  - Hayward Gallery
  - National Theatre
  - Oxo Tower
  - Purcell Room
  - Queen Elizabeth Hall
  - Royal Festival Hall
  - Shakespeare's Globe
  - Tate Modern
- ▶ Speakers' Corner
- ▶ St Bartholomew-the-Great
- ▶ St Martin-in-the-Fields
- ▶ St Paul's Cathedral
  - Golden Gallery
  - Whispering Gallery
- ▶ Temple
  - Temple Church
- ▶ Tower Bridge
- ▶ Tower of London
  - Beefeaters
  - Crown Jewels
- ▶ Trafalgar Square
- ▶ Wembley Stadium
- ▶ West End
- ▶ Westminster Abbey
- ▶ Westminster Bridge
- ▶ Westminster Cathedral
- ▶ Whitehall
- ▶ Wilton's Music Hall
- ▶ Windsor Castle
- ▶ Ye Olde Cheshire Cheese Pub

LONDON: TOP MUSEUMS

▶ British Museum
▶ Charles Dickens Museum
▶ Churchill War Rooms
▶ Freud Museum
▶ Geffrye Museum
▶ Imperial War Museum
▶ Leighton House Museum
▶ London Transport Museum
▶ Museum of London
▶ National Maritime Museum
▶ Natural History Museum
▶ Science Museum
▶ Sherlock Holmes Museum
▶ Sir John Soane's Museum
▶ Victoria and Albert Museum
▶ Wellcome Collection

LONDON: TOP GALLERIES

▶ Apsley House
▶ Courtauld Gallery
▶ Dulwich Picture Gallery
▶ Hayward Gallery
▶ National Gallery
▶ National Portrait Gallery
▶ Royal Academy of Arts
▶ Tate Britain
▶ Tate Modern
▶ Wallace Collection

LONDON: TOP PARKS

▶ Green Park
▶ Hampstead Heath

- Keats House
- Kenwood House
▶ Holland Park
  - Kyoto Garden
▶ Hyde Park
  - Serpentine Lake
▶ Kensington Gardens
▶ Regent's Park
  - Open Air Theatre
▶ Richmond Park
▶ Royal Botanic Gardens Kew
▶ St James's Park

LONDON: TOP VIEWS

▶ Hampstead Heath
  - Parliament Hill Fields
▶ London Eye
▶ Monument
▶ Oxo Tower
▶ Royal Observatory
▶ Shard
▶ Sky Garden
▶ Tower Bridge

LONDON: TOP SHOPPING

▶ Bond Street
▶ Burlington Arcade
▶ Camden Market
▶ Carnaby Street
▶ Covent Garden
▶ Jermyn Street
▶ Kings Road
▶ Leadenhall Market
▶ Marylebone High Street

► Old Spitalfields Market

► Old Truman Brewery

► Oxford Street

► Portobello Market

► Savile Row

► Westfield Shopping Centre

LONDON: TOP SHOPS

► Asprey: Jewellery

► Barnard & Westwood: Printing

► Berry Bros. & Rudd: Wine

► Boodles: Jewellery

► Crocket & Jones: Shoes

► Ettinger: Leatherware

► Floris: Perfume

► Fortnum & Mason: Retail

► Foster & Son: Shoes

► Foyles: Books

► Gieves & Hawkes: Clothing

► Harrods: Retail

► Harvie & Hudson: Shirts

► Hatchards: Books

► Henry Poole & Co: Clothing

► Huntsman: Suits

► John Lobb: Shoes

► Liberty: Fashion

► Lock & Co: Hats

► Paxton & Whitfield: Cheese

► Selfridges: Retail

► Smythson: Stationery

► Thomas Goode & Co: Tableware

► Thresher & Glenny: Clothing

► Turnbull & Asser: Shirts

► Twinings: Tea

NORTHERN ENGLAND: TOP ATTRACTIONS

▶ Berwick-upon-Tweed
▶ Blackpool
▶ Chester
  • Rows
▶ Durham
  • Castle
▶ Fountains Abbey and Studley Royal Water Garden
▶ Hadrian's Wall
  • Housesteads
▶ Haworth
▶ Lake District
  • Grasmere
  • Windermere
▶ Leeds
  • Kirkgate Market
  • Leeds Art Gallery
  • Leeds Corn Exchange
  • Leeds Town Hall
  • River Aire
  • Royal Armouries Museum
▶ Liverpool
  • Albert Dock
    ▪ Museums
▶ Manchester
  • Castlefield
  • John Rylands Library
  • Manchester Art Gallery
  • Museum of Science and Industry
  • Old Trafford
  • Salford Quays
    ▪ Imperial War Museum North
    ▪ Lowry
    ▪ MediaCityUK
  • Spinningfields
  • Town Hall

► Newcastle
- Discovery Museum
- Grainger Town
- Millennium Bridge
► Peak District
- Bakewell
- Buxton
- Castleton
► Saltaire
► Whitby
► York
- Jorvik Viking Centre
- National Railway Museum
- Shambles
- York Minster
► Yorkshire Dales
- Richmond

CENTRAL ENGLAND: TOP ATTRACTIONS

► Birmingham
- Birmingham Museum and Art Gallery
- Canals
- Symphony Hall
► Cambridge
- Backs
- King's College
- Pepys Library
- Trinity College
- Wren Library
► Cotswolds
- Berkeley
- Bibury
- Bourton-on-the-Water
- Broadway
- Burford

- Castle Combe
- Cheltenham
- Chipping Campden
- Cirencester
- Gloucester
- Painswick
- Stow-on-the-Wold
- Tewkesbury
- The Slaughters
- Winchcombe
▶ Leicester
▶ Lincoln
▶ Nottingham
▶ Oxford
  - Ashmolean Museum
  - Bodleian Library
  - Christ Church College
  - Magdalen College
  - Radcliffe Camera
▶ Shropshire
  - Ironbridge Gorge
▶ Stratford-upon-Avon
  - Anne Hathaway's Cottage
  - Holy Trinity Church
  - Royal Shakespeare Theatre
  - Shakespeare's Birthplace
▶ Warwick

SOUTHWEST ENGLAND: TOP ATTRACTIONS

▶ Avebury
▶ Bath
  - Bath Abbey
  - Circus
  - Georgian Garden
  - Pulteney Bridge

▶ Stonehenge

▶ Wells

SOUTHEAST ENGLAND: TOP ATTRACTIONS

▶ Brighton
  - Brighton Pavilion
  - Brighton Pier
▶ Canterbury
  - Canterbury Cathedral
▶ Colchester
▶ Isle of Wight
▶ Kent
▶ New Forest
▶ Norfolk
▶ Portsmouth
▶ Suffolk
▶ Winchester
  - Winchester Cathedral

ENGLAND: TOP CASTLES AND STATELY HOMES

▶ Bedfordshire
  - Luton Hoo
  - Woburn Abbey
▶ Berkshire
  - Highclere Castle
▶ Cheshire
  - Lyme Park
▶ Derbyshire
  - Chatsworth House
  - Crag Hall
  - Hardwick Hall
▶ Gloucestershire
  - Sudeley Castle
▶ Hampshire
  - Beaulieu

▶ Hertfordshire
  • Hatfield House
▶ Kent
  • Hever Castle
  • Leeds Castle
▶ Lincolnshire
  • Burghley House
▶ London
  • Kenwood House
▶ Norfolk
  • Blickling Hall
  • Holkham Hall
▶ Oxfordshire
  • Blenheim Palace
  • Buscot Park
  • Stonor
▶ Somerset
  • Montacute House
▶ Suffolk
  • Somerleyton Hall
▶ Warwickshire
  • Warwick Castle
▶ Wiltshire
  • Great Chalfield Manor
  • Lacock Abbey
  • Longleat House
  • Stourhead
▶ Yorkshire
  • Castle Howard
  • Harewood House
  • Norton Conyers
  • Wentworth Woodhouse

EDINBURGH: TOP ATTRACTIONS

▶ Arthur's Seat
▶ Calton Hill

- City Observatory
- National Monument
- Nelson Monument
► Camera Obscura
► Charlotte Square
► Edinburgh Castle
  - Great Hall
  - Military Tattoo
  - Royal Palace
► George Heriot's School
► George Street
► Grassmarket
► Greyfriars Bobby
► Greyfriars Church
► John Knox House
► National Museum of Scotland
► National Portrait Gallery
► Palace of Holyroodhouse
  - The Queen's Gallery
► Port of Leith
  - Firth of Forth
  - Forth Rail Bridge
  - Royal Yacht Britannia
► Portobello Beach
► Princes Street
  - Princes Street Gardens
  - Scott Monument
► Queen Street
► Rosslyn Chapel
► Royal Botanic Garden
► Royal Mile
  - Canongate
  - Castle Hill
  - High Street
  - Lawnmarket
► Royal Scottish Academy
► Scottish National Gallery

► Scottish Parliament

► St Giles' Cathedral

► Stockbridge

SCOTLAND: TOP ATTRACTIONS

► Aberdeen
  • Old Aberdeen
► Ben Nevis
► Culloden Battlefield
► Culzean Castle
► Eilean Donan Castle
► Fort William
► Glamis Castle
► Glasgow
  • Gallery of Modern Art
  • Kelvingrove Art Gallery and Museum
  • People's Palace
  • Riverside Museum
► Glen Coe
► Grampian Mountains
► Inner Hebrides
  • Isle of Iona
  • Isle of Mull
  • Isle of Skye
► Inverness
► John O'Groats
► Loch Ness
► Northwest Highlands
  • Wildlife
► Oban
► Orkney Islands
  • Skara Brae
► Outer Hebrides
► Perthshire
  • Scone Palace

- ▶ Royal Deeside
  - • Balmoral Castle
  - • Braemar Castle
- ▶ Shetland Islands
- ▶ Speyside
  - • Whisky
- ▶ St Andrews
  - • Golf
- ▶ Stirling
  - • Stirling Castle
  - • Wallace Monument
- ▶ Trossachs
  - • Loch Katrine
  - • Loch Lomond
- ▶ Urquhart Castle

CARDIFF: TOP ATTRACTIONS

- ▶ Bute Park
- ▶ Cardiff Bay
- ▶ Cardiff Castle
- ▶ Mermaid Quay
- ▶ National Assembly for Wales
- ▶ National Museum Cardiff
- ▶ Wales Millennium Centre
- ▶ Wales Millennium Stadium

WALES: TOP ATTRACTIONS

- ▶ Anglesey
- ▶ Brecon Beacons
- ▶ Caernarfon Castle
- ▶ Gower Peninsula
- ▶ Llandudno
- ▶ Pembrokeshire
  - • St Davids

457

- ▶ Porthmadog
- ▶ Portmeirion
- ▶ Snowdonia
  - • Betws-y-Coed
  - • Capel Curig
  - • Dolgellau
  - • Snowdon
- ▶ Tintern Abbey

BELFAST: TOP ATTRACTIONS

- ▶ Belfast Castle
- ▶ Botanical Gardens
- ▶ City Hall
- ▶ Crown Liquor Saloon
- ▶ Grand Opera House
- ▶ Parliament Buildings
- ▶ Queen's University
- ▶ Titanic Belfast
- ▶ Ulster Museum
- ▶ Waterfront

NORTHERN IRELAND: TOP ATTRACTIONS

- ▶ Ards Peninsula
- ▶ Armagh
- ▶ Causeway Coastal Route
- ▶ Derry
- ▶ Enniskillen Castle
- ▶ Giant's Causeway
- ▶ Lough Erne
- ▶ Mourne Mountains
- ▶ Ulster American Folk Park
- ▶ Ulster Folk and Transport Museum

BRITONS

GREAT BRITONS

▶ Adam Smith – Economist

▶ Alan Turing – Computer scientist

▶ Alec Guinness – Actor

▶ Alexander Graham Bell – Telephone

▶ Alfred Hitchcock – Film director, film producer

▶ Benjamin Disraeli – Conservative politician

▶ Captain James Cook – Explorer

▶ Charles Darwin – Biologist, evolution

▶ Charlie Chaplin – Actor, film director, comedian

▶ Christopher Cockerell – Hovercraft

▶ Christopher Wren – St Paul's Cathedral

▶ David Attenborough – Naturalist

▶ David Livingstone – Explorer

▶ Edward Jenner – Smallpox vaccine

▶ Edwin Lutyens – Architect

▶ Emmeline Pankhurst – Suffragette

▶ Ernest Shackleton – Explorer

▶ Florence Nightingale – Nursing reformer

▶ Francis Drake – Explorer

▶ Frank Whittle – Jet engine

▶ George Fox – Quaker

▶ George Stephenson – Steam locomotive

▶ Henry Hudson – Explorer

▶ Henry Wood – Conductor

▶ Hugh Grant – Actor

▶ Inigo Jones – Architect

▶ Isaac Newton – Gravitation, mechanics, motion

▶ Isambard Kingdom Brunel – Engineer

▶ James Dewar – Thermos flask

▶ James Goodfellow – Cash machine

▶ James Hargreaves – Spinning Jenny

▶ James Watt – Steam engine

- ▶ John Dalton – Atomic theory
- ▶ John Logie Baird – Television
- ▶ John Maynard Keynes – Economist
- ▶ John Wesley – Methodism
- ▶ Josiah Wedgwood – Pottery
- ▶ Lancelot Capability Brown – Landscape architect
- ▶ Laurence Olivier – Actor
- ▶ Margaret Rutherford – Actress
- ▶ Michael Faraday – Diamagnetism, electromagnetic induction, electrolysis
- ▶ Nicholas Grimshaw – Architect
- ▶ Norman Foster – Architect
- ▶ Richard Arkwright – Carding machine
- ▶ Richard Burton – Actor
- ▶ Richard Rogers – Architect
- ▶ Robert Falcon Scott – Explorer
- ▶ Robert Watson-Watt – Radar
- ▶ Samuel Pepys – Diary
- ▶ Sean Connery – Actor
- ▶ Stephen Hawking – Theoretical cosmology, quantum gravity
- ▶ Terence Conran – Designer
- ▶ Thomas Chippendale – Furniture
- ▶ Thomas Edward Lawrence – Lawrence of Arabia
- ▶ Tim Berners-Lee – World Wide Web
- ▶ Walter Bagehot – The Economist
- ▶ Walter Raleigh – Explorer
- ▶ William Beveridge – Social insurance
- ▶ William Booth – Salvation Army
- ▶ William Caxton – Printer
- ▶ William Ewart Gladstone – Liberal politician
- ▶ William Wilberforce – Philanthropist
- ▶ Winston Churchill – Statesman

BRITISH

GREAT BRITISH ATTITUDES AND MANNERS

- ▶ Adhering to the rules
- ▶ Apologising needlessly
- ▶ Avoiding confrontation
- ▶ Awareness of history
- ▶ Class consciousness
- ▶ Coded speech
- ▶ Common sense
- ▶ Consciousness of tradition
- ▶ Courtesy
- ▶ Decency
- ▶ Down to earth
- ▶ Eccentricity
- ▶ Fair play
- ▶ Forming a queue
- ▶ Imperturbability
- ▶ Individualism
- ▶ Irony
- ▶ Keeping a stiff upper lip
- ▶ Love of liberty
- ▶ Moderation
- ▶ Modesty
- ▶ Not showing off
- ▶ Patriotism
- ▶ Politeness
- ▶ Pragmatism
- ▶ Punning
- ▶ Rationality
- ▶ Refusing to complain
- ▶ Relationship with nature
- ▶ Reserve
- ▶ Respect
- ▶ Saying sorry

- ▶ Self deprecation
- ▶ Self discipline
- ▶ Sense of humour
- ▶ Sense of identity
- ▶ Sportsmanship
- ▶ Stoicism
- ▶ Talking about the weather
- ▶ Team spirit
- ▶ Understatement
- ▶ Willingness to compromise

GREAT BRITISH SYMBOLS AND INSTITUTIONS

- ▶ 10 Downing Street
- ▶ Afternoon tea
- ▶ Aston Martin
- ▶ Bagpipes
- ▶ Balmoral Castle
- ▶ Barbour jacket
- ▶ Barrister's wig
- ▶ Bed and Breakfast
- ▶ Belisha beacon
- ▶ Betting
- ▶ Bingo
- ▶ Black cab
- ▶ Black humour
- ▶ Bobby
- ▶ Bowler hat
- ▶ Braemar Gathering
- ▶ British Airways
- ▶ British Army
- ▶ British Broadcasting Corporation
- ▶ Buckingham Palace
- ▶ Bulldog
- ▶ Burberry coat
- ▶ Canals

- ► Cardigan
- ► Carnaby Street
- ► Castles
- ► Cathedrals
- ► Ceremonies
- ► Ceremony of the Keys
- ► Changing of the Guard
- ► Charities
- ► Chelsea Flower Show
- ► Chequers
- ► Christmas cracker
- ► City of London
- ► Clubs
- ► Cockney
- ► Comedy
- ► Committees
- ► Concorde
- ► Cool Britannia
- ► Corgi
- ► 'Coronation Street'
- ► Countryside
- ► Cowes Week
- ► Crown Jewels
- ► 'Dad's Army'
- ► Dartboard
- ► Deckchair
- ► Deerstalker
- ► 'Doctor Who'
- ► Dress codes
- ► 'EastEnders'
- ► Edinburgh International Festival
- ► 'Emmerdale'
- ► Eton College
- ► Fleet Street
- ► Flying Scotsman
- ► Fortnum & Mason

- ▶ Garden gnome
- ▶ Garden shed
- ▶ Gentleman
- ▶ Gilbert and Sullivan operas
- ▶ Glyndebourne Festival
- ▶ Guy Fawkes Night
- ▶ Harrods
- ▶ Heathrow Airport
- ▶ Henley Royal Regatta
- ▶ Highland Games
- ▶ HMS Victory
- ▶ Hogmanay
- ▶ Honours
- ▶ Hot and cold taps
- ▶ Hunting pink
- ▶ Imperial units
- ▶ Jaguar
- ▶ James Bond
- ▶ John Bull
- ▶ Kilt
- ▶ King Arthur
- ▶ King James Bible
- ▶ Landscape garden
- ▶ Last Night of the Proms
- ▶ London Tube map
- ▶ Lord's Cricket Ground
- ▶ Mini
- ▶ 'Monty Python's Flying Circus'
- ▶ Most Noble Order of the Garter
- ▶ National Health Service
- ▶ National Trust
- ▶ Nessie
- ▶ Notting Hill Carnival
- ▶ Old Bailey
- ▶ Old Boys' Club
- ▶ Old Trafford

- ▶ Oxbridge
- ▶ Oxford and Cambridge Boat Race
- ▶ Oxford English Dictionary
- ▶ Oyster card
- ▶ Palace of Holyroodhouse
- ▶ Pantomime
- ▶ Pets
- ▶ Policeman's helmet
- ▶ Pound Sterling
- ▶ Pub
- ▶ Public footpaths
- ▶ Range Rover
- ▶ Red pillar box
- ▶ Red telephone box
- ▶ Remembrance Day
- ▶ Remembrance poppy
- ▶ Right of way
- ▶ Robin Hood
- ▶ Rolls-Royce
- ▶ Routemaster bus
- ▶ Royal Academy Summer Exhibition
- ▶ Royal Air Force
- ▶ Royal and Ancient Golf Club
- ▶ Royal Ascot
- ▶ Royal Edinburgh Military Tattoo
- ▶ Royal Mail
- ▶ Royal Marsden Hospital
- ▶ Royal Military Academy Sandhurst
- ▶ Royal Navy
- ▶ Royalty
- ▶ Sandringham House
- ▶ School uniform
- ▶ Scotland Yard
- ▶ Seaside resorts
- ▶ Selfridges
- ▶ Spitfire

- ▶ 'Spitting Image'
- ▶ State Opening of Parliament
- ▶ Swan upping
- ▶ Tartan
- ▶ Teapot
- ▶ Terraced houses
- ▶ Thames
- ▶ Thatched cottages
- ▶ 'The Archers'
- ▶ 'The Economist'
- ▶ 'The Spectator'
- ▶ 'The Times'
- ▶ Three-pin plug
- ▶ Titanic
- ▶ Trench coat
- ▶ Trooping the Colour
- ▶ Tube
- ▶ Tweed jacket
- ▶ Underdog
- ▶ Union Jack
- ▶ Wellington boots
- ▶ Wembley Stadium
- ▶ West End
- ▶ Westminster Abbey
- ▶ White Cliffs of Dover
- ▶ Wimbledon tennis
- ▶ Windsor Castle
- ▶ Winnie-the-Pooh
- ▶ 'Yes Minister'

GREAT BRITISH PROVERBS AND IDIOMS

- ▶ A bad penny always turns up.
- ▶ A friend in need is a friend indeed.
- ▶ Actions speak louder than words.
- ▶ All that glitters is not gold.

- ▶ Always have sunshine in your heart.
- ▶ Always look on the bright side.
- ▶ An apple a day keeps the doctor away.
- ▶ Bad news travels fast.
- ▶ Better late than never.
- ▶ Brevity is the soul of wit.
- ▶ Desperate situations call for desperate measures.
- ▶ Don't let it get you down.
- ▶ Easier said than done.
- ▶ Easy come, easy go.
- ▶ Every cloud has a silver lining.
- ▶ Every little helps.
- ▶ Fine words butter no parsnips.
- ▶ Fingers crossed.
- ▶ Go the extra mile.
- ▶ Great minds think alike.
- ▶ Home is where the heart is.
- ▶ Honesty is the best policy.
- ▶ If a job's worth doing, it's worth doing well.
- ▶ Imitation is the sincerest form of flattery.
- ▶ In for a penny, in for a pound.
- ▶ It'll be all right.
- ▶ It's not as bad as it seems.
- ▶ It's not cricket.
- ▶ Jack of all trades is master of none.
- ▶ Keep calm and carry on.
- ▶ Keep the flag flying.
- ▶ Knowledge is power.
- ▶ Laugh and the world laughs with you.
- ▶ Life goes on.
- ▶ Little things please little minds.
- ▶ Live and let live.
- ▶ Mind your own business.
- ▶ My home is my castle.
- ▶ No news is good news.
- ▶ No pain, no gain.

- ▶ Now the ball is in your court.
- ▶ One does what one can.
- ▶ One gets used to anything.
- ▶ Out of sight, out of mind.
- ▶ That could happen to anyone.
- ▶ That's the way it is.
- ▶ The devil is in the detail.
- ▶ The early bird catches the worm.
- ▶ The exception proves the rule.
- ▶ The grass is always greener on the other side of the fence.
- ▶ The situation is hopeless, but not serious.
- ▶ There's no place like home.
- ▶ Things always seem worse than they are.
- ▶ Things don't always turn out as expected.
- ▶ This is not rocket science.
- ▶ Time flies.
- ▶ Time is a great healer.
- ▶ Times have changed.
- ▶ To err is human, to forgive divine.
- ▶ Tomorrow is another day.
- ▶ We will take it as it comes.
- ▶ What can go wrong, will go wrong.
- ▶ When the cat's away, the mice will play.
- ▶ Where there's a will, there's a way.
- ▶ Who knows what the point of it all is.
- ▶ You can't do anything about it.
- ▶ You can't have your cake and eat it too.
- ▶ You can't know everything.
- ▶ You can't take it with you.
- ▶ You have to move with the times.
- ▶ You never know.

BUSINESS PHRASES

CHAPTER OVERVIEW

- DECIDING
- CLOSING
- MISCELLANEOUS
▶ MINUTES
  - PHRASES FOR MINUTES
  - STATING
  - CITING
▶ REPORTS
  - PHRASES FOR REPORTS
  - CONTENT
  - FEATURES
  - ANALYSIS
  - COMMENT
  - PARALLELS
  - CONTRASTS
  - SUPPORT
  - QUESTIONING
  - DISAPPROVAL
  - CONCLUSION
▶ PUBLICATIONS
  - PHRASES FOR PUBLICATIONS
  - INTRODUCTION
  - METHODS
  - RESULTS
  - DISCUSSION
  - CONCLUSION
  - ACKNOWLEDGEMENT
▶ PRESENTATIONS
  - PHRASES FOR PRESENTATIONS
  - PROBLEMS
  - STARTING
  - SETTING
  - OVERVIEW
  - SEGUE
  - CHARTS
  - GRAPHS

- ENDING
- FAREWELL
► MODERATION
  - PHRASES FOR MODERATION
  - INTRODUCTION
  - DISCUSSION
  - CONTENT
  - QUALITY
  - VOTE
  - TIME
  - ADJOURNMENT
  - DIGRESSION
  - IMPOLITENESS
► CORRESPONDENCE
  - PHRASES FOR CORRESPONDENCE
  - STARTING
  - REQUESTING
  - REMINDING
  - CONFIRMING
  - REGRETTING
  - APPRECIATING
  - INVITING
  - MEETING
  - CANCELLING
  - INFORMING
  - HELPING
  - THANKING
  - MISCELLANEOUS
  - ENDING
► PHONECALLS
  - PHRASES FOR PHONECALLS
  - STARTING
  - TROUBLESHOOTING
  - BRIDGING
  - ACTING
  - ASKING

- **ADVISING**
- **REFLECTING**
- **HELPING**
- **GREETING**
- **MISCELLANEOUS**
- **THANKING**
- **REPLYING**
- **APOLOGISING**
- **REACTING**
- **ENDING**

MEETINGS

PHRASES FOR MEETINGS

▶ Show genuine interest.
▶ Ask open questions.
▶ Keep the ball rolling.
▶ Always mind your manners.

▶ Come to the point, make your point, keep to the point.
▶ Use plain language, use common words, use short sentences.
▶ Be clear, be straight, be fair.

ENQUIRING

▶ When would suit you …
▶ When are you free …
▶ When would be convenient …

REPLYING

▶ Confirming
  - That would be fine …
  - I look forward to …

▶ Declining
- Sorry, but I will not be available then …
- I am afraid I am busy that day/am tied up then/cannot manage that day …
- Sorry, but I unfortunately have another engagement on …

▶ Changing
- Is there any chance we could move the meeting …
- I am afraid I need to change the date …

▶ Cancelling
- Due to limited resources I regret that I will not be able to attend the meeting …

INVITING

▶ I would like to invite you to …

▶ Enclosed (letter)/attached (email) is a participant list and our provisional agenda …

▶ The event is taking place on … at …

▶ If you have any comments or further suggestions, please let me know …

▶ Could you kindly confirm your attendance by …

INTRODUCING

▶ Introduction
- I don't think we've met before. My name is …
- May I introduce myself? I am …
- I don't think we've been introduced. My name is …

▶ Reply
- Pleased to meet you. My name is …
- How do you do? I am …
- Nice to meet you. My name is …

OPENING

▶ Shall we begin/get down to business/get started …

WELCOMING

▶ More formal
  - I have the honour to declare ... open ...
  - On behalf of ... please allow me to extend to you a very warm welcome ...
  - I feel honoured to welcome you to ...
▶ More informal
  - It is a pleasure to welcome you ...
  - I am glad you could make it ...

COMMENCING

▶ Have all participants seen the minutes of the last meeting ...
▶ Who is taking the minutes today ...
▶ I circulated the agenda in advance ...
▶ We can start with the first item on the agenda ...

GOALSETTING

▶ The aim/objective/purpose of this discussion/meeting/negotiation is ...
  - What we need to deal with is ...
  - I have called a meeting to ...
  - What we should address/consider/discuss is ...
  - The reason for coming together is ...
  - What we ought to find out is ...

PROPOSING

▶ Making proposals
  - I would like to suggest that we add to the agenda ...
  - I think we should also take up the issue/problem/question of ...
  - I would like to propose that we remove from the agenda ...
▶ Resisting proposals
  - I am sorry but I do not think ...
  - I suggest we confine ourselves to ...
  - We will probably not have the time to ...

▶ Modifying proposals

- I believe the point you have suggested is already covered by ...
- Perhaps we should rather consider the issue of ... in conjunction with ...

CONVERSING

▶ Information

- I would like to learn more about ...
- Could you please be more specific about ...
- Could you please expand on this point ...
- I think we need more details about ...

▶ Clarification

- I did not catch your point ...
- Would you mind explaining it again ...
- What exactly do you mean by ...
- Could you go over it again ...
- Am I correct in assuming that ...

▶ Paraphrase

- I am sorry for the confusion ...
- In other words ...
- Let me put it another way ...
- The point I am trying to make is ...
- What I wish to say is ...
- In specific terms ...
- Does this all make sense now ...

▶ Expansion

- Other aspects to consider are ...
- Another thought which occurs to me is ...
- I should also refer to ...

▶ Return

- As I have mentioned before ...
- Could we go back to ...

▶ Opinion

- What are your impressions about ...
- I would like to invite you to present your views on ...
- May I ask you for your comments/thoughts/views on ...

- I was just wondering if you would like to comment on …
- How do you feel about …

REASONING

▶ Starting
- I would like to share with you some thoughts on …
- As far as I know/to my knowledge …
- If I am not mistaken …
- It seems to me that …
- For my part/in my judgement/in my mind/in my opinion/in my view …
- If I remember this rightly …
- I might be wrong but …
- In my experience/so far as I remember …
- I would like to raise a number of questions about …

▶ Developing
- This leads me to the point that …
- I should like to draw attention to/point out/put emphasis on/single out …
- I would now like to move to …

▶ Illustrating
- Take, for example, …
- Let me illustrate this point …
- I should also mention that …
- I would like to make this clear by means of an example …
- I mention this in passing …
- A case in point is …
- Take, for instance, …

▶ Comparing
- Let me draw a comparison …
- This case is similar to ours …
- Let me compare this with …

▶ Stressing
- At the outset, it should be clearly understood that …
- I hold the firm view that …
- It is my clear contention that …
- I would like to emphasise/highlight/reiterate/stress/underline/underscore …

- No sensible person can deny that …
- Every sensible person will agree on …
- In my view, there can be no doubt that …

▶ Questioning
- The question has to be asked whether …
- The reasoning is flawed/problematic/questionable …
- This gives rise to some fundamental difficulties …

▶ Balancing
- Although …, I nevertheless think …
- We need to consider …
- We need to recognise …
- We need to remember …
- However …
- Yet …
- On the one hand …, on the other hand …
- Nonetheless …
- Nevertheless …
- We should not forget …
- We should not ignore …
- We should not overlook …
- While …, there is evidence …

▶ Qualifying
- In all fairness …
- With all due care …
- Without wishing to offend anyone …
- We should do justice to both sides …
- Without wishing to give offence …
- With all due caution …
- To be fair …

▶ Summarising
- All in all …
- In a word …
- In conclusion …
- The quintessence …
- On balance …
- So much for …
- To sum up …

AGREEING

▶ Strong agreement
- I agree with …
- I am strongly convinced that …
- I accept without any hesitation …
- It goes without saying that …
- I am at one with you …
- I had a very similar experience to what …
- … deserves our entire/full/wholehearted backing/endorsement/support …
- I was once in exactly the same situation …
- I simply must agree with you …
- It stands to reason that …
- I am in agreement with …
- I am in favour of …
- I endorse that …

▶ Weak agreement
- I basically/principally agree but …
- By and large …
- With certain reservations …
- I think along the same lines but …
- I am inclined to agree with … but …
- In a sense …
- In a way …
- I could/would agree but …

DISAGREEING

▶ Strong disagreement
- Quite the contrary …
- Quite the opposite …
- I absolutely disagree with …
- I am in disagreement with …
- Under no circumstances will I agree to …
- It is absolute nonsense to think that …
- You commit a serious error …

- We differ completely on this point …
- On the contrary …
- You are really jumping to conclusions …
- You cannot be taken seriously …
- It is utterly wrong to believe that …
- I cannot but reject this proposal outright …
- What I object to is …
- I am decidedly against …
- By no means …
- Far from it …

► Weak disagreement

- I would rather say that …
- I am not quite sure but …
- I do not share your view …
- What makes you say that …
- That is not necessarily so …
- I understand what you are saying but …
- If you see the matter from another angle …
- I am not convinced/persuaded by …
- If you look at it from another angle …
- There is more to it than that …
- This is not strictly true …
- It is quite debatable that …
- I really cannot agree with you …
- I see it a little differently …
- I tend to think that …

REAFFIRMING

► We cannot ignore …

► It is safe to say that …

► We should not lose sight of …

► We have no option but to …

► It is absolutely out of the question …

► I would even go so far as to say that …

► It is crucial/essential/imperative/vital that we bear in mind/keep in mind/take into account/take into consideration …

- As everyone knows, … is by far the most important aspect …
- You can take my word for it …
- This is undoubtedly in keeping with …
- I need to say once more …
- It is an accepted fact that …
- Let me repeat …

DOUBTING

- I am sceptical about …
- I am still not sure that …
- Even so, we ought to ask ourselves whether …
- These standpoints cannot be compared …
- This idea/notion/proposal/suggestion has some contradictions/limitations/ shortcomings/weaknesses …
- These views are incompatible with …
- This does not rule out the fact that …
- It is open to question whether …
- I seriously doubt that …

OBJECTING

- Despite …, I am still convinced that …
- I take a different view on …
- This argument misses the point …
- The fact is that …
- The criticisms made/objections raised fail to consider/recognise …
- The fact remains that …
- We are obviously divided on …
- In contrast to what you said …
- Thank you for raising this, but …

INTERRUPTING

- Making an interruption
  - I am very sorry to interrupt you but …

- If I may come in at this point …
- Before you go any further, I would like …
- Could I just say a few words about …
▶ Managing an interruption
  - With your permission, I would like to finish what I was saying …
  - If you would allow me to finish off first …
  - Please bear with me for a moment, I shall be dealing with your point a little later …
  - Coming back to what I was trying to explain …
  - Thank you for your comment, I will come back to you shortly …

DELAYING

▶ I think we should look at this issue more carefully …
▶ Perhaps we should deal with … first …
▶ I feel a decision at this stage would be premature …

REASSURING

▶ Do not worry …
▶ Please rest assured …
▶ You may be confident …
▶ Everything in my power will be done …
▶ You have my word …
▶ I assure you …
▶ I promise you …

INSISTING

▶ I have decided …
▶ My decision is final …
▶ I made up my mind …
▶ You cannot change my mind anymore …
▶ I shall on no account …
▶ I will not accept …
▶ I am determined …

REVISING

▶ I take it all back …

▶ I must admit I was wrong …

▶ I have made a mistake …

BARGAINING

▶ We might be able to solve this issue if …

▶ I could agree with … provided that …

▶ If you could accept …, I would be willing to …

CONCEDING

▶ After careful consideration, I am persuaded that …

▶ Your objection is justified …

▶ I must admit that the points you made have convinced me …

▶ I did not consider …

▶ Your arguments are so persuasive that I …

COMPROMISING

▶ It seems as if we could all agree on …

▶ In my view, a fair compromise would be …

▶ If we consider both sides …

▶ The following compromise is conceivable …

▶ Both sides now agree on …

▶ Can we reach agreement along the following lines …

▶ We have found common ground in so far as …

CONCLUDING

▶ If I may go over the main points we have heard …

▶ I think we can draw the following conclusions from our discussion …

▶ I would like to summarise the most compelling arguments as follows …

DECIDING

▶ We have agreed that …
▶ It is settled then that …
▶ We have decided that …

CLOSING

▶ Is there anything else you wish to add …
▶ I would like to draw this meeting to a close …
▶ I would like to thank everyone for their excellent contributions …
▶ I think that completes our agenda for today …

MISCELLANEOUS

▶ Really good to see you again …
▶ Let's have dinner sometime …
▶ Do you happen to know …
▶ Can I just make a point …
▶ I'll let you know first thing tomorrow morning …
▶ I'm happy we got that out of the way …
▶ I'll be in touch with you again soon …
▶ Just a second, before I forget …
▶ Now you must excuse me …
▶ See you again soon …
▶ It was good talking to you …

MINUTES

PHRASES FOR MINUTES

▶ Come to the point, make your notes, keep to the point.
▶ Use plain language, use common words, use short sentences.
▶ Be correct, be objective, be specific.

STATING

▶ He/she
- accentuated …
- accepted …
- acknowledged …
- adapted …
- added …
- admitted …
- admonished …
- advised …
- advocated …
- agreed …
- announced …
- anticipated …
- appealed …
- approved …
- argued …
- asked …
- asserted …
- assumed …
- attempted …
- believed …
- caused …
- cautioned …
- checked …
- cited …
- claimed …
- commented …
- compared …
- conceded …
- concluded …
- confirmed …
- confused …
- conjectured …
- considered …

- contended ...
- convinced ...
- correlated ...
- debated ...
- decided ...
- declared ...
- declined ...
- deduced ...
- demonstrated ...
- denied ...
- depicted ...
- described ...
- detected ...
- discussed ...
- disproved ...
- documented ...
- elucidated ...
- emphasised ...
- encouraged ...
- endorsed ...
- enquired ...
- envisaged ...
- estimated ...
- evidenced ...
- expected ...
- explained ...
- expressed ...
- falsified ...
- felt ...
- found ...
- guessed ...
- highlighted ...
- identified ...
- illustrated ...
- implied ...
- indicated ...

- induced …
- inferred …
- informed …
- insisted …
- intended …
- investigated …
- judged …
- maintained …
- mentioned …
- noted …
- objected …
- observed …
- opposed …
- pinpointed …
- portrayed …
- postulated …
- praised …
- precluded …
- predicted …
- presented …
- presumed …
- pretended …
- promised …
- proposed …
- proved …
- purported …
- quantified …
- quoted …
- recalled …
- recognised …
- recommended …
- recorded …
- recounted …
- remained …
- remarked …
- reminded …

- repeated …
- replied …
- reported …
- reproduced …
- required …
- revealed …
- said …
- screened …
- searched …
- showed …
- solved …
- speculated …
- stated …
- strengthened …
- stressed …
- suggested …
- supported …
- supposed …
- suspected …
- tested …
- told …
- tried …
- underlined …
- underscored …
- urged …
- varied …
- verified …
- warned …
- welcomed …
- wondered …
- worked …

CITING

▶ To cite …
▶ In the words of …

▶ With reference to …

▶ … made a case against/in favour of …

▶ The text at hand is taken from …

▶ With regard to …

▶ According to the text …

▶ To quote …

REPORTS

PHRASES FOR REPORTS

▶ Accounts

▶ Reports

▶ Reviews

CONTENT

▶ The author
- argues against …
- calls into question …
- makes us aware of …
- attaches great attention to …
- puts forward the thesis that …
- contradicts/criticises/questions …
- falsifies/formulates/verifies a hypothesis …
- expounds his/her thoughts about …
- sets out his/her ideas on …
- expresses/utters/voices his/her opinion/view about …
- furnishes/produces/provides his/her evidence/proof of …
- points out his/her attitude towards …
- outlines his/her position on …
- disproves/proves/rejects an argument …
- accuses/blames/condemns …
- comments on the situation that …
- takes into consideration that …

- contradicts the statement about …
- is canvassing for …
- protests against …

▶ The text

- The central/main/principal message …
- Addresses/appeals to/argues that/begins with/comprises/concludes with/consists of/constitutes/deals with/divides into/ends with/explains/expresses/interprets/is about/is composed of/is divided into/is intended for/is made up of/reflects/reveals/says that/shows/starts with …
- The grounds/motive/reason for …

FEATURES

▶ Assertive/concise/factual/informative/logical text

- … has a favourable/high/positive opinion about …
- … has a low/negative/unfavourable opinion about …
- … expresses his/her respect for/satisfaction with/sympathy for …
- … expresses his/her antipathy towards/aversion to/dislike of …
- … shows a low/reasonable/special interest in …
- … displays an intimate/superficial/thorough knowledge of …

▶ Ambiguous/animated/clear/colloquial/complicated/dated/direct/elevated/formal/impersonal/restrained/simple/vague/vivid language

▶ Humorous/ironic/sarcastic/serious/technical tone

ANALYSIS

▶ I would like to explore this point further …

▶ It is generally accepted/assumed/known that …

▶ I must not fail to mention that …

▶ This argument is not a convincing one …

▶ There has been controversy/debate/discussion about …

▶ I have to take a closer look at …

COMMENT

▶ Fortunately/happily …

▶ Regrettably/unfortunately …

- ▶ Presumably/probably …
- ▶ Inevitably/necessarily …
- ▶ It is certain/clear/evident/notable/noticeable/obvious/remarkable/proven …
- ▶ Interestingly/remarkably …
- ▶ Demonstrably/obviously …
- ▶ Predictably/typically …
- ▶ Amazingly/surprisingly …

PARALLELS

- ▶ This also extends to …
- ▶ This also refers to …
- ▶ There are parallels between …
- ▶ The points have in common …
- ▶ The following similarities are apparent …
- ▶ As a rule/for the most part/generally/in principle/in the main/normally/on the whole/usually …
- ▶ We concur in the following …
- ▶ The same is true for …
- ▶ There is consistency among …
- ▶ This applies equally to …
- ▶ This is similar to …

CONTRASTS

- ▶ However …
- ▶ While …
- ▶ In comparison with …
- ▶ Contrary to which …
- ▶ In contrast to …
- ▶ On the contrary …
- ▶ As opposed to …
- ▶ Conversely …
- ▶ Unlike …

SUPPORT

▶ A convincing/plausible/powerful/solid argument for …

▶ The author carries conviction in the statement that …

▶ There can be no doubt that …

▶ I am delighted to read that …

▶ The text is groundbreaking/impartial/interesting/profound …

▶ It is likely/obvious/probable/true …

▶ The article is balanced/informative/insightful/objective …

▶ It is with great pleasure that …

▶ The author quite rightly states that …

▶ The author is certainly correct in saying that …

▶ A conclusive/crucial/decisive/important reason for …

QUESTIONING

▶ It is not possible to accept this assertion as it stands …

▶ On the other hand …

▶ The arguments are greatly disputed/highly questionable/not compelling/too superficial/very doubtful …

▶ However, some contradictions arise …

▶ This appears to be a valid argument only at first glance …

DISAPPROVAL

▶ It is an indefensible/misleading/untenable argument that …

▶ It is unimaginable/unlikely/unthinkable that …

▶ I am unable to share this view …

▶ I refute this view …

▶ I reject this argument …

▶ The text contains many factual/linguistic errors …

▶ This statement is completely wrong …

▶ The report is biased/manipulative/meaningless/unimaginative/unsubstantiated …

▶ The opposite is the case …

▶ The article has been poorly/superficially researched …

▶ I am disappointed with …

▶ I am shocked by …
▶ The objection can be made here that …
▶ It seems disputable/questionable/uncertain that …
▶ It is an unfounded/unsubstantiated/untrue assertion that …

CONCLUSION

▶ With all due caution …
▶ It has become apparent that …
▶ It has clearly emerged that …
▶ After carefully weighing up all the facts …
▶ In view of all these facts …
▶ The long and the short of it is …
▶ All things considered/in a nutshell/in brief/in essence/in short/in summary/overall/summarising …
▶ To put the whole matter in a nutshell …
▶ Contrary to the generally held view …
▶ The facts permit only the following conclusion …
▶ I arrive at the conclusion …
▶ The conclusion I may draw …
▶ I have just shown …

PUBLICATIONS

PHRASES FOR PUBLICATIONS

▶ Academic papers
▶ Scientific papers

INTRODUCTION

▶ Subject
  • Analysis/article/report/review/study/survey
▶ Aim
  • Aim/focus/goal/intent/objective/purpose

METHODS

▶ To address/to analyse/to assess/to attempt/to compare/to describe/
to determine/to evaluate/to examine/to explore/to illustrate/to intend/
to investigate/to measure/to monitor/to observe/to perform/to present/to
process/to report/to retrieve/to review/to screen/to test

RESULTS

▶ Finding/outcome/result
▶ Frequency/incidence/rate
▶ To range from … to …/to vary from … to …
▶ To detect/to identify/to reveal
▶ To demonstrate/to indicate/to show

DISCUSSION

▶ Mentioning
  ● To consider/to detect/to disclose/to encounter/to mention/to name/to
    observe/to perceive/to report/to reveal
▶ Describing
  ● To delineate/to depict/to describe/to illustrate/to scrutinise/to specify
▶ Comparing
  ● With regard to/with respect to
  ● In accordance with/in agreement with/in keeping with/in line with
  ● To deviate from/to differ from/to disagree with/to vary from
  ● To correlate with/to correspond with
▶ Analysing
  ● Consequently/hence/therefore/thus
  ● Depending on/subject to
  ● Attributable to/because of/due to/owing to
  ● To come from/to originate from/to result from/to stem from
  ● Independent of/irrespective of/regardless of/separate from
  ● Along with/together with
  ● Detailed/exhaustive/extensive/thorough
▶ Emphasising
  ● Considerable/critical/crucial/essential/important/impressive/paramount/
    particular/significant/special/striking/vital

▶ Interpreting
  - To confirm/to corroborate/to prove/to support
  - To be associated with/to be based on/to be related to
  - To disapprove/to disprove/to object/to reject

CONCLUSION

▶ As a consequence/as a result/consequently/finally/in conclusion/to summarise

ACKNOWLEDGEMENT

▶ To address thanks/to express gratitude/to extend thanks/to owe gratitude
  - For advice/assistance/help/support

PRESENTATIONS

PHRASES FOR PRESENTATIONS

▶ Lectures
▶ Speeches
▶ Talks

PROBLEMS

▶ Unfortunately, I do not know how this device works …
▶ Where can I find the light switch …
▶ I cannot access my computer file …
▶ There is an error message …
▶ The … does not function/work …
▶ Do you have an adapter …
▶ I need an extension cord for …
▶ Can I plug in my laptop somewhere …
▶ How can I attach the projector to my computer …

STARTING

▶ Thank you for your warm welcome …

▶ It is my pleasure to be here with you …

▶ I would like to express my sincere gratitude to … for inviting me to …

▶ I am most grateful to … for inviting me to …

▶ Thank you for the kind welcome …

SETTING

▶ The whole presentation will probably take about … minutes …

▶ Please ask your questions as soon as they arise …

▶ I apologise for this brief interruption, we can carry on in a second …

▶ There will be ample time for discussion at the end of the presentation …

▶ I will answer all your questions at the end …

▶ I will distribute a handout after the presentation …

OVERVIEW

▶ The focus of my presentation is …

▶ I have divided the presentation as follows …

▶ I will be covering the following aspects/issues/items/problems/subjects …

▶ In this context I will look at …

▶ I would like to concentrate on …

SEGUE

▶ I will now move on to …

▶ This brings me to the next point …

▶ These issues are important for the next point …

▶ The next slides are related to this aspect …

▶ This leads me to a different issue …

▶ I want to go on with …

CHARTS

▶ Area chart
▶ Bar chart
▶ Flow chart
▶ Line chart
▶ Organisational chart
▶ Pie chart
▶ Tree chart
  • Diagonal/horizontal/vertical axis
  • Broken/dotted/solid line

GRAPHS

▶ The diagram shows …
▶ These figures convey a clear message …
▶ I would like to draw your attention to this chart in particular …
▶ I base this statement particularly on …
▶ The statistics support …

ENDING

▶ Thank you for your kind attention …
▶ I have now come to the end of my presentation …
▶ Allow me to summarise the basic facts …
▶ Let me run through the main arguments again …
▶ Let us go over the main points again …
▶ Allow me now to make an assessment …
▶ I do hope my presentation sheds a different light on …
▶ Thank you very much for listening …

FAREWELL

▶ Thank you for your attention …
▶ I hope you enjoyed it …
▶ Thank you for being here …

MODERATION

PHRASES FOR MODERATION

- ▶ Keep calm.
- ▶ Put the speakers at ease.
- ▶ Stay on top of things.
- ▶ Retain control.

INTRODUCTION

- ▶ I would like to welcome you all here to …
- ▶ I have the great pleasure of introducing …
- ▶ … will now speak to you about the problem of …

DISCUSSION

- ▶ I would welcome any questions and comments …
- ▶ Does anyone else wish to take the discussion further …
- ▶ Let me pass this question to … who is an expert on this matter …
- ▶ I suggest leaving this point aside for the moment …
- ▶ Thank you very much for your interest …

CONTENT

- ▶ Please stick to facts …
- ▶ Please consider this objectively …
- ▶ I do not know what to make of this …
- ▶ I think that is a matter of opinion …
- ▶ These remarks should not go without comment …
- ▶ What are the most convincing arguments for that claim …
- ▶ This individual case cannot be transferred quite so simply …
- ▶ You cannot simply deduce a universal rule from this …
- ▶ We should treat this point in detail …
- ▶ You cannot simply shrug off such a problem …
- ▶ I cannot make any sense of what … is saying …

▶ Where is the evidence …

▶ What counts here is …

QUALITY

▶ What I liked particularly was …

▶ You have hit the nail on the head in saying …

▶ I have really enjoyed your excellent presentation …

▶ What you were saying is beside the point …

▶ I think your presentation was very useful …

▶ The quality of your presentation leaves much to be desired …

▶ What I did not understand …

VOTE

▶ Could we take a vote on this …

- Who is in favour …
- Those against …
- Are there any abstentions …

▶ The proposal is hereby accepted/rejected …

▶ The objection is hereby accepted/overruled …

▶ The voting has resulted in a tie …

▶ The motion has been carried unanimously …

▶ Irrespective of which side one takes …

▶ The participants are divided on the subject …

TIME

▶ Please keep it short …

▶ We need to go on …

▶ We are running behind schedule …

▶ Could you keep your comment short …

▶ Pardon me for interrupting you but …

▶ We are running out of time …

▶ We are going over time …

▶ Please observe the time limit …

▶ Our time is limited …

ADJOURNMENT

▶ We will have a short break …

▶ The session is adjourned until …

▶ The session will resume in …

▶ Thank you all for your participation …

DIGRESSION

▶ This is of no importance …

▶ This is of no significance …

▶ I need to intervene at this point …

▶ This is moving away from the topic at hand …

▶ We should go back to the core of the matter …

▶ That has nothing to do with what we are discussing …

▶ I am afraid we are moving away from the subject …

▶ This is not even remotely related to our topic …

▶ We should rather return to the topic …

▶ What really matters here is …

▶ Please keep to the point …

IMPOLITENESS

▶ Personal criticism will most definitely not help us here …

▶ Please avoid getting personal, and stick to the issues …

▶ I am sorry, but you are being offensive …

▶ We should also let the others get a word in …

▶ I am sorry, but you are becoming rude …

▶ Sorry, this is not going to get us anywhere …

▶ I do not think we should go into this …

CORRESPONDENCE

PHRASES FOR CORRESPONDENCE

▶ Emails
▶ Letters

▶ Use a logical structure.
▶ Use paragraphs.
▶ Use a clear layout.

▶ Write active sentences.
▶ Write meaningful sentences.
▶ Write positive sentences.
▶ Write short sentences.

▶ Be authentic.
▶ Be clear.
▶ Be concise.
▶ Be confident.
▶ Be direct.
▶ Be inclusive.
▶ Be passionate.
▶ Be positive.
▶ Be professional.
▶ Be visionary.

▶ Avoid catchphrases.
▶ Avoid clichés.
▶ Avoid exaggeration.
▶ Avoid jargon.
▶ Avoid redundancy.
▶ Avoid vagueness.

STARTING

▶ I was delighted to get your letter …

▶ Thank you very much for your letter of …

▶ I appreciate your interest and thank you for writing to me …

▶ I was pleased to hear from you again …

▶ I was glad to get your reply …

▶ I hope you are well …

▶ Just a note to inform you …

▶ I am writing to ask about/confirm that/enquire about/inform you …

▶ This is to notify you of …

▶ I trust everything is fine …

▶ With reference to …

▶ Referring to …

▶ … as agreed/discussed/indicated/requested …

▶ Further to …

▶ In reply to …

▶ On the basis of your …

▶ Subject to …

▶ Should this be the case, please …

▶ Depending on …

▶ From what you write about …

▶ I am happy to announce …

▶ I would like to bring to your attention that …

▶ It gives me great pleasure to inform you that …

  • I enclose …

  • Please find attached/enclosed …

    ▪ Please note from the attached documents that …

  • The enclosed …

▶ I take this opportunity to …

▶ I have forwarded your letter to …
▶ I have passed it on to …

▶ I note with surprise that …
▶ I write to express my concern …
▶ Could you please explain to me why you …
▶ I must confess to feeling annoyed at the tone of your letter …
▶ I demand an explanation from you as to …
▶ I consider this to be inappropriate …
▶ I fail to understand why …

REQUESTING

▶ I would appreciate it if …
▶ I would like to …
▶ Could you please …
▶ Would you mind just …
▶ Would you be good enough to …
▶ Could you kindly answer these questions …
▶ I therefore request that …
▶ I wonder if …
▶ I am interested in …
▶ I would be grateful if …
  • I hope for an early reply …
  • I would be grateful if you could deal with this matter as soon as possible/at your earliest convenience …
    ▪ I need it within …
    ▪ I need it by …
    ▪ I do not need it until …
    ▪ I need it before …
    ▪ I need it on …
  • Please deal with this matter urgently …

REMINDING

- ▶ I was wondering if you had had time to …
- ▶ I know that you are extremely busy, but could you possibly …
- ▶ I am just writing to …
- ▶ Did you get my last message, sent on …
- ▶ Given that I have not heard from you, I am worried that I did not explain the issue clearly …
- ▶ As you can see from the attached emails below, I have in fact raised this issue several times before …
- ▶ May I remind you that I am still …
- ▶ Just a quick reminder that …
- ▶ I am sorry to bother you again, but I urgently need …
- ▶ I would just like to remind you of/that …

CONFIRMING

- ▶ I acknowledge receipt of your letter of …
- ▶ I confirm our meeting which was scheduled at … on …
- ▶ I am looking forward to your acknowledgement/confirmation …
- ▶ I would like to confirm the appointment at … on …
- ▶ I am delighted/happy/pleased to confirm …

REGRETTING

- ▶ I am writing to apologise for missing the deadline …
- ▶ I am sorry to hear that …
- ▶ Unfortunately, I am unable …
- ▶ Much to my regret …
- ▶ I do wish I could give you a more satisfactory answer …
- ▶ I regret that I am unable to give you a more favourable reply …
- ▶ Please accept my apologies for any inconvenience this has caused you …
- ▶ With great regret, I …
- ▶ Regretfully, I have decided …
- ▶ I regret to inform you that …
- ▶ I am afraid that I have to tell you …

APPRECIATING

▶ Please accept my sincere appreciation for all the kind assistance and help you gave me in ...

▶ Without you and your professional team, this success would not have been possible ...

▶ I have been pleased with the exceptional service of you and your team ...

▶ I very much appreciate your assistance in solving these difficult matters, and I look forward to ...

INVITING

▶ Invitation
  • Allow me to invite you ...
  • May I invite you ...
  • I cordially invite you to ...

▶ Positive response
  • Thank you very much ..., I am looking forward to ...
  • Thank you very much for your invitation to ..., which I will be happy to attend ...
  • Thank you very much ..., I would love to come ...

▶ Negative response
  • I am afraid I cannot make it ...
  • I sincerely regret that I am unable to accept the invitation because of another engagement/due to a prior commitment ...
  • I am sorry but I have to ...

▶ Politeness
  • Just a short note to thank you again for a most enjoyable evening ...
  • I do hope you will give me an opportunity to return your hospitality ...

MEETING

▶ When would it be convenient for you to meet with me ...

▶ I would be willing to meet you at any time at your convenience to ...

▶ Please drop me a line as to when we could meet ...

CANCELLING

- ▶ Unfortunately, I have to inform you that I cannot keep our appointment on …
- ▶ Much to my regret, I have to cancel …
- ▶ Thank you very much for your understanding …
- ▶ I would suggest we postpone our meeting until …
- ▶ Please let me know if this date is convenient for you or if …

INFORMING

- ▶ I will keep you updated …
- ▶ I will contact/get back to/get in touch with/inform/notify/send you …
- ▶ I will let you know …

HELPING

- ▶ Please contact me if you have any questions …
- ▶ Please inform me about any difficulties or problems …
- ▶ Please feel free to mail me any queries …
- ▶ If you have any more questions, please do not hesitate to contact me …
- ▶ Should you need any further information, I will be happy to assist you …
- ▶ If you would like any more details, please let me know any time …

THANKING

- ▶ Thank you in advance for your help …
- ▶ I would like to express my thanks to you for …
- ▶ Thank you for all the trouble you went to on my behalf …
- ▶ Thank you for the confidence you have shown in me …
- ▶ Thank you once again for your assistance …

MISCELLANEOUS

- ▶ It is my policy to …
- ▶ I set great store by …

- ▶ According to what you told me about …
- ▶ I cannot rule out the possibility that …
- ▶ I would have wished for something different …
- ▶ I will, unfortunately, have no alternative but to …
- ▶ I would welcome an explanation as to why …
- ▶ I hope you will appreciate that I must …
- ▶ This is due entirely to circumstances beyond my control …
- ▶ There is always something turning up to prevent me from …
- ▶ I think I did not express myself quite clearly there …
- ▶ I am sorry I cannot give you any information about that …
- ▶ I am afraid I do not want to express an opinion on the matter …
- ▶ And with that, I would like to draw a line under this particular point …
- ▶ I am very sorry to give you such short notice and I sincerely hope that this …
- ▶ I am confident that we will be able to clarify the matter to our mutual satisfaction …
- ▶ I must ask you to make sure that/solve this problem/take prompt action …
- ▶ Please accept in advance my great thanks for any help you can give me …
- ▶ Should I not hear from you to the contrary, I will …
- ▶ I will need some more time to think about it …
- ▶ I will, of course, leave this entirely to your discretion …
- ▶ We should also be prepared for the fact that …
- ▶ This statement has proved/turned out to be …
- ▶ It is virtually out of the question that …
- ▶ I cannot tell you yet whether or not …
- ▶ I should like to remind you that …
- ▶ I am unfortunately compelled/forced/obliged to …
- ▶ Please let me have your comments on …
- ▶ I shall refrain from doing …
- ▶ I am not entitled to …

ENDING

- ▶ Thank you again for your kindness …
- ▶ Just give me a ring if …
- ▶ Please keep me in the loop …
- ▶ I look forward to your response …

▶ I would be delighted to hear from you …
▶ I hope to hear from you again soon …
▶ I look forward to hearing from you soon …
▶ I hope to stay in touch with you …

PHONECALLS

PHRASES FOR PHONECALLS

▶ Formal phone calls
▶ Informal phone calls

STARTING

▶ Could I speak to …, please …
▶ I would like to have a word with …
▶ Is this a good time for you to …
▶ I just wanted to give you a quick call …
▶ Could you please connect me with/put me through to …
▶ I will not take up much of your time …
▶ Could you spare me a few moments, please …
▶ I am phoning you about a serious matter …
▶ Shall I call back later …

▶ Thank you very much, I will hold …
▶ I cannot hold any longer …
▶ I think I will ring again later …
▶ When would suit you best …

▶ Could you call me back …
▶ Could you ask … to phone me back …
▶ Could you perhaps leave a message for …
▶ Thanks for returning my call …

- ▶ I am phoning to …
- ▶ I am calling to ask you …
- ▶ I hope I am not disturbing you …
- ▶ Would you be so kind as to …
- ▶ I am ringing to inform you …
- ▶ I would like to …

- ▶ I am sorry to keep you waiting …
- ▶ I will be with you right away …

- ▶ Thank you for calling but …
- ▶ I am short of time …
- ▶ Sorry, but I am in a meeting …
- ▶ Unfortunately, I am very busy at the moment …
- ▶ Sorry, but I have to finish now …
- ▶ I am in a hurry …
- ▶ I will call you back …

TROUBLESHOOTING

- ▶ Pardon …
- ▶ Sorry, I did not get …
- ▶ I did not quite catch that …
- ▶ I cannot follow what you are saying …
- ▶ I am sorry I missed your call …
- ▶ I will transfer you back to …
- ▶ Would you please repeat that …
- ▶ Sorry …

BRIDGING

- ▶ Last time we talked …
- ▶ Talking about our plans …
- ▶ I will pick up where we left off last time …

▶ If I remember right …

▶ That reminds me of …

ACTING

▶ I am currently in the process of …

▶ I am arranging/due/likely/planning to …

▶ I have in the meantime spoken to …

ASKING

▶ I was wondering if I might ask …

▶ Could you give me any information on …

▶ Can you recall/remember …

▶ I would like some more information about …

▶ I wonder if you could tell me …

ADVISING

▶ What do you advise me to do …

▶ I would like to hear your opinion …

▶ What would you do if you were in my place …

▶ If you want my opinion …

▶ I would strongly advise you …

REFLECTING

▶ I will think about it …

▶ I have not made up my mind yet …

▶ I am not sure yet …

HELPING

▶ I will get it sorted out now …

▶ I will check that for you …

- ▶ I will look into this immediately …
- ▶ I will work it out for you …
- ▶ Can you leave it with me …
- ▶ I will take care of it …
- ▶ I will be doing everything possible to …

GREETING

- ▶ Please give my regards to …
- ▶ Remember me to …
- ▶ Please convey my best wishes to …
- ▶ Best wishes to …
- ▶ Say hello to … from me …

MISCELLANEOUS

- ▶ We seem to be talking at cross purposes …
- ▶ Am I right in assuming that …
- ▶ Could you make this enquiry in writing, please …
- ▶ Could you confirm that in writing, please …
- ▶ Please mark the envelope 'for the attention of' …
- ▶ Could you do me a favour …
- ▶ With respect, that is not what I said …

THANKING

- ▶ I am grateful for your kind assistance …
- ▶ Thank you very much indeed, that is very kind of you …
- ▶ Thank you for having been so helpful …

REPLYING

- ▶ Don't mention it …
- ▶ Not at all …
- ▶ Don't worry about it …

▶ It's no trouble at all …

▶ It was my pleasure …

▶ That's all right …

▶ You're very welcome …

APOLOGISING

▶ I'm afraid that …

▶ I really must apologise …

▶ I did not mean it this way …

▶ Please accept my apologies for the inconvenience caused …

▶ I am sorry not to be of any further help …

▶ That was not my intention. I will look into the matter immediately. The mistake will be rectified as soon as possible …

▶ I hope we will be able to arrange something else …

▶ This was due to circumstances beyond my control …

▶ I think there has been a misunderstanding …

▶ Please accept my apologies …

▶ I'm sorry that …

REACTING

▶ That's okay …

▶ It doesn't matter …

▶ That's all right …

▶ No need to apologise …

▶ These things happen …

▶ No harm done …

▶ Never mind …

ENDING

▶ This was all the information I needed …

▶ Thank you for calling …

▶ I think that's it for now …

▶ It has been nice talking to you …

▶ I will talk to you later/soon …

▶ I will get back to you soon …

▶ I guess that's all for now …

▶ Have a nice day …

▶ Thank you and all the very best …

ESSENTIAL GRAMMAR

CHAPTER OVERVIEW

▶ **GRAMMAR**
▶ **CONDITIONAL CLAUSE**
▶ **REPORTED SPEECH**
▶ **SUBJUNCTIVE**

GRAMMAR

▶ The English language is a cultural treasure and full of beauty.

▶ Spelling, punctuation and grammar are essential for mastering the English language.

▶ The English language is a veritable minefield and full of pitfalls.

CONDITIONAL CLAUSE

▶ Real conditional clause in the present and future
  • Present tense → Future tense

▶ Unreal conditional clause in the present and future
  • Past tense → Would + infinitive

▶ Unreal conditional clause in the past
  • Past perfect → Would have + past participle

REPORTED SPEECH

▶ Present simple → Past simple
▶ Present progressive → Past progressive
▶ Present perfect simple → Past perfect simple

513

- ▶ Present perfect progressive → Past perfect progressive
- ▶ Past simple → Past perfect simple
- ▶ Past progressive → Past perfect progressive
- ▶ Future simple → Conditional simple
- ▶ Future progressive → Conditional progressive
- ▶ Future perfect simple → Conditional perfect simple
- ▶ Future perfect progressive → Conditional perfect progressive

- ▶ Going to-future → Was/were going to

- ▶ I/you/we/you → He/she/they
- ▶ My/your/our/your → His/her/their
- ▶ Here → There
- ▶ This → That
- ▶ These → Those
- ▶ Now → Then
- ▶ Ago → Before
- ▶ The day before yesterday → Two days before
- ▶ Yesterday → The day before/the previous day
- ▶ Today → That day
- ▶ Tomorrow → The following day/the next day
- ▶ The day after tomorrow → In two days' time

- ▶ Can → Could
- ▶ May → Might
- ▶ Shall → Should
- ▶ Will → Would

- ▶ Must → Must (conclusion, prohibition, rule)/had to (obligation, near future)/ would have to (obligation, distant future)
- ▶ Must not → Must not (conclusion, prohibition, rule)/was/were not allowed to
  - • I must not → I was not to
- ▶ Need → Need
- ▶ Need not → Did not have to/would not have to

SUBJUNCTIVE

▶ Sentences which do not describe known objective facts

▶ State of mind

- Belief
- Desire
- Intention
- Opinion
- Purpose

▶ Following these verbs

- To demand
- To insist
- To propose
- To recommend
- To suggest

▶ Infinitive without to

- Examples
  - She suggested that he examine the patient …
  - She suggested that the patient be admitted …

BIBLIOGRAPHY

► Abib-Pech, Marianne | Leadership
► Academy of Medical Royal Colleges | A framework of principles for mentoring
► Academy of Medical Royal Colleges | Appraisal for revalidation – A guide to the process
► Academy of Medical Royal Colleges | Choosing wisely
► Academy of Medical Royal Colleges | Core principles for continuing professional development
► Academy of Medical Royal Colleges | Global health capabilities for UK health professionals
► Academy of Medical Royal Colleges | Medical careers – A flexible approach in later years
► Academy of Medical Royal Colleges | Quality improvement – Training for better outcomes
► Academy of Medical Royal Colleges | Standards for the clinical structure and content of patient records
► Academy of Medical Royal Colleges | Supporting information for appraisal and revalidation
► Academy of Medical Royal Colleges | Workforce
► Academy of Medical Royal Colleges, NHS Institute for Innovation and Improvement | Medical leadership competency framework
► Academy of Medical Royal Colleges, NHS Institute for Innovation and Improvement | Medical leadership curriculum
► Acas | Building productivity in the UK
► Acas | Bullying and harassment at work – A guide for employees
► Acas | Bullying and harassment at work – A guide for managers and employers
► Acas | Challenging conversations and how to manage them
► Acas | Code of practice on disciplinary and grievance procedures
► Acas | Conducting workplace investigations
► Acas | Discipline and grievances at work
► Acas | Discrimination – What to do if it happens
► Acas | Equality and discrimination – Understand the basics

▶ Acas | Health, work and wellbeing

▶ Acas | How to manage change

▶ Acas | How to manage performance

▶ Acas | Managing anxiety in the workplace

▶ Acas | Managing attendance and employee turnover

▶ Acas | Managing conflict at work

▶ Acas | Managing people

▶ Acas | Managing staff absence

▶ Acas | Model workplace

▶ Acas | New to HR – Helpful Acas resources for you

▶ Acas | Prevent discrimination – Support equality

▶ Acas | Productivity tool

▶ Acas | Promoting positive mental health in the workplace

▶ Acas | Recruiting staff

▶ Acas | Starting staff – Induction

▶ Acas | Stress at work

▶ Acas | Top tips for better management

▶ Acas | Workplace trends

▶ Aggarwal, Reena; Swanwick, Tim | Clinical leadership development in postgraduate medical education and training – Policy, strategy, and delivery in the UK National Health Service

▶ Armstrong, Michael | How to be an even better manager

▶ Baldoni, John | The leader's guide to speaking with presence

▶ Barr, Jill; Dowding, Lesley | Leadership in health care

▶ Bell, Andrew | Employment law

▶ Bevan, Aneurin | In place of fear – A free health service

▶ Bowden, Michelle | How to present

▶ Bradberry, Travis; Greaves, Jean | Leadership 2.0

▶ British Medical Association, NHS Employers | Good rostering guide

▶ Britnell, Mark | In search of the perfect health system

▶ Bucci, Ronald | Medicine and business

▶ Burnison, Gary | The leadership journey

▶ Care Quality Commission | Celebrating good care, championing outstanding care

▶ Care Quality Commission | Complaints matter

▶ Care Quality Commission | Driving improvement

▶ Care Quality Commission | Enforcement action and representations

▶ Care Quality Commission | Guidance for providers

▶ Care Quality Commission | How CQC regulates

▶ Care Quality Commission | How we do our job

▶ Care Quality Commission | How we inspect and regulate – A guide for providers

▶ Care Quality Commission | Inspection framework

▶ Care Quality Commission | Inspection reports

▶ Care Quality Commission | Learning, candour and accountability

▶ Care Quality Commission | Learning from serious incidents in NHS acute hospitals

▶ Care Quality Commission | Planning the inspection

▶ Care Quality Commission | Quality improvement in hospital trusts – Sharing learning from trusts on a journey of QI

▶ Care Quality Commission | Ratings

▶ Care Quality Commission | Registering and monitoring services

▶ Care Quality Commission | Regulations for service providers and managers

▶ Care Quality Commission | Requesting a review of ratings

▶ Care Quality Commission | Review of CQC's impact on quality and improvement in health and social care

▶ Care Quality Commission | Safeguarding people

▶ Care Quality Commission | Shaping the future

▶ Care Quality Commission | State of care

▶ Care Quality Commission | Supporting information and guidance – Qualifications and continuing professional development requirements for registered managers and for the practitioners they supervise

▶ Care Quality Commission | Supporting information and guidance – Supporting effective clinical supervision

▶ Care Quality Commission | Taking action

▶ Care Quality Commission | The five key questions we ask

▶ Care Quality Commission | The fundamental standards

▶ Care Quality Commission | The state of care in independent acute hospitals

▶ Care Quality Commission | The state of care in NHS acute hospitals

▶ Care Quality Commission | The state of care in urgent primary care services

▶ Care Quality Commission | What can you expect from a good hospital?

▶ Care Quality Commission | What to expect when we inspect

▶ Care Quality Commission | What we do on an inspection

▶ Carnegie, Dale | How to win friends and influence people

▶ Carr, Claudia | Beginning medical law

▶ Carroll, John | Effective project management

▶ Carroll, John | Effective time management

▶ Chartered Institute of Personnel and Development | Job-seeking guides

▶ Chartered Institute of Personnel and Development | Manage your career

▶ Chartered Institute of Personnel and Development | Organisational culture and behaviours

▶ Chartered Institute of Personnel and Development | People management fundamentals

▶ Chartered Institute of Personnel and Development | Strategy and planning

▶ Coburn, Calum | Negotiation styles

▶ Committee on Standards in Public Life | The 7 principles of public life

▶ Commonwealth Fund | Mirror, mirror

▶ Covey, Stephen | The 7 habits of highly effective people

▶ Dale, Iain | The NHS – Things that need to be said

▶ Day, Gary; Leggat, Sandra | Leading and managing health services – An Australasian perspective

▶ Department of Health | An NHS we love to work for

▶ Department of Health | A promise to learn – A commitment to act

▶ Department of Health | Better leadership for tomorrow – NHS leadership review

▶ Department of Health | Change4Life

▶ Department of Health | High quality care for all – NHS next stage review final report

▶ Department of Health | Improving NHS staff engagement

▶ Department of Health | NHS mandate

▶ Department of Health | NHS outcomes framework – At-a-glance

▶ Department of Health | NHS staff management and health service quality

▶ Department of Health | Operational productivity and performance in English NHS acute hospitals – Unwarranted variations

▶ Department of Health | Report of the Mid Staffordshire NHS Foundation Trust public inquiry

▶ Department of Health | The government's mandate to NHS England

▶ Department of Health | The health and care system explained

▶ Department of Health | The health and social care act

▶ Department of Health | The NHS choice framework – What choices are available to me in the NHS?

▶ Department of Health | The role of the responsible officer

▶ Department of Health | Your NHS care – Changing your hospital

▶ Department of Health | Your NHS care – Choosing your hospital

▶ Department of Health, NHS Commissioning Board | Compassion in practice

▶ Dhamija, Bhoresh; Keane, Margaret; Low, Chen Sheng; Ghosh, Robert | Clinical audit for doctors and healthcare professionals

▶ Dillon, Henry; Sandison, George | Life in the UK study guide

▶ Dorling Kindersley | Achieving high performance

▶ Dorling Kindersley | Leadership

▶ Dorling Kindersley | Managing people

▶ Dorling Kindersley | Negotiating

▶ Dorling Kindersley | Project management

▶ Dorling Kindersley | The business book

▶ Dorling Kindersley | The essential managers handbook

▶ Douglas, Neil | Improving medical leadership

▶ Duckworth, Angela | Grit – The power of passion and perseverance

▶ Faculty of Medical Leadership and Management | Building resilience – A practical resource for healthcare professionals

▶ Faculty of Medical Leadership and Management | Developing medical leadership

▶ Faculty of Medical Leadership and Management | Leadership and leadership development in health care – The evidence base

▶ Faculty of Medical Leadership and Management | Leadership and management standards for healthcare teams

▶ Faculty of Medical Leadership and Management | Leadership and management standards for medical professionals

▶ Faculty of Medical Leadership and Management | Leading as a junior doctor

▶ Faculty of Medical Leadership and Management | Medical leadership and management – An indicative undergraduate curriculum

▶ Faculty of Medical Leadership and Management | Supporting information for appraisal and revalidation – Speciality guidance for the leadership and management aspects of a doctor's scope of practice

▶ Faculty of Medical Leadership and Management | The state of medical leadership and management training for junior doctors

▶ Faculty of Medical Leadership and Management | Transitions – Clinical director

▶ Faculty of Medical Leadership and Management | Transitions – Medical chief executive

▶ Faculty of Medical Leadership and Management | Transitions – Medical director

▶ Faculty of Medical Leadership and Management, NHS Improvement | The medical director induction guide – Supporting recently appointed medical directors

▶ Faculty of Medical Leadership and Management, NHS Providers, NHS Improvement | Eight high impact actions to improve the working environment for junior doctors

▶ Ferlie, Ewan; Montgomery, Kathleen; Pedersen, Anne | The Oxford handbook of health care management

▶ Fox, Jeffrey | How to become CEO – The rules for rising to the top of any organisation

► Francke, Ann | Management

► General Medical Council | A guide for doctors reported to the GMC

► General Medical Council | A guide for health professionals on how to report a doctor to the GMC

► General Medical Council | Confidentiality – Good practice in handling patient information

► General Medical Council | Consent – Patients and doctors making decisions together

► General Medical Council | Continuing professional development – Guidance for all doctors

► General Medical Council | Delegation and referral

► General Medical Council | Effective governance to support medical revalidation – A handbook for boards and governing bodies

► General Medical Council | Generic professional capabilities framework

► General Medical Council | Good medical practice

► General Medical Council | Good medical practice framework for appraisal and revalidation

► General Medical Council | Guidance for doctors acting as responsible consultants or clinicians

► General Medical Council | Guidance for doctors – Requirements for revalidation and maintaining your licence

► General Medical Council | Guidance on supporting information for appraisal and revalidation

► General Medical Council | Guidance to doctors working under system pressure

► General Medical Council | How to complain about a doctor

► General Medical Council | Leadership and management for all doctors

► General Medical Council | Openness and honesty when things go wrong – The professional duty of candour

► General Medical Council | Raising and acting on concerns about patient safety

► General Medical Council | The GMC protocol for making revalidation recommendations

► General Medical Council | The reflective practitioner – Guidance for doctors and medical students

► General Medical Council | The state of medical education and practice in the UK

► General Medical Council | Writing references

► George, Bill | True north – Discover your authentic leadership

► George, Mike; Rowlands, Dave; Kastle, Bill | What is lean six sigma?

► Godbole, Prasad; Burke, Derek; Aylott, Jill | Why hospitals fail

► Goleman, Daniel | Emotional intelligence – Why it can matter more than IQ

▶ Good Governance Institute | A simple guide to risk for members of boards and governing bodies

▶ Good Governance Institute | Complaints handling in NHS organisations

▶ Good Governance Institute | Diversity – The new prescription for the NHS

▶ Good Governance Institute | Good governance in European healthcare – The NHS in England

▶ Good Governance Institute | How population health management will deliver a sustainable NHS

▶ Good Governance Institute | NHS trust board good governance maturity matrix

▶ Good Governance Institute | The future of the NHS

▶ Good Governance Institute | The role of the medical director in the NHS

▶ Good Governance Institute | What every healthcare director needs to know about patient safety

▶ Goodall, Amanda; Stoller, James | The future of clinical leadership – Evidence for physician leadership and the educational pathway for new leaders

▶ Gopee, Neil; Galloway, Jo | Leadership and management in healthcare

▶ Gottwald, Mary; Lansdown, Gail | Clinical governance – Improving the quality of healthcare for patients and service users

▶ Guest, Charles; Ricciardi, Walter; Kawachi, Ichiro; Lang, Iain | Oxford handbook of public health practice

▶ Habicht, Robert; Gulati, Mangla | Hospital medicine

▶ Harvard Business Essentials | Manager's toolkit

▶ Harvard Business Review | Be a better boss

▶ Harvard Business Review | Building a workforce for the future

▶ Harvard Business Review | Diversity

▶ Harvard Business Review | How to be a good board chair

▶ Harvard Business Review | How to work with toxic colleagues

▶ Harvard Business Review | Management tips

▶ Harvard Business Review | Managing time

▶ Harvard Business Review | On managing across cultures

▶ Harvard Business Review | Seven transformations of leadership

▶ Hasson, Gill | Mindfulness pocketbook

▶ Health Education England | Leadership development for doctors in postgraduate medical training

▶ Health Education England | Leadership for clinicians

▶ Health Foundation | A practical guide to self-management support

▶ Health Foundation | Continuous improvement of patient safety

▶ Health Foundation | Evaluation – What to consider

▶ Health Foundation | Healthy lives for people in the UK

▶ Health Foundation | How does the NHS compare with health systems in other countries?

▶ Health Foundation | Leading in a crisis – The power of transparency

▶ Health Foundation | New approaches to value in health and care

▶ Health Foundation | NHS at 70 – How good is the NHS?

▶ Health Foundation | NHS at 70 – Public perceptions

▶ Health Foundation | Person-centred care made simple

▶ Health Foundation | Quality improvement made simple

▶ Health Foundation | Simpler, clearer, more stable – Integrated accountability for integrated care

▶ Health Foundation | The spread challenge – How to support the successful uptake of innovations and improvements in health care

▶ Health Foundation | Using communication approaches to spread improvement

▶ Health Foundation | What makes us healthy?

▶ Health Foundation | What the system can do

▶ Healthcare Financial Management Association | Emerging approaches – Developing sustainability and transformation plan governance arrangements

▶ Healthcare Financial Management Association | Glossary for NHS and local government finance and governance

▶ Healthcare Improvement Scotland | Driving improvement in the quality of healthcare

▶ Healthcare Quality Improvement Partnership | Best practice in clinical audit

▶ Healthcare Quality Improvement Partnership | Clinical audit – A guide for NHS boards and partners

▶ Healthcare Quality Improvement Partnership | Developing a clinical audit policy

▶ Healthcare Quality Improvement Partnership | Developing a clinical audit programme

▶ Healthcare Quality Improvement Partnership | Developing a clinical audit strategy

▶ Healthcare Quality Improvement Partnership | Documenting local clinical audit – A guide to reporting and recording

▶ Healthcare Quality Improvement Partnership | Good governance handbook

▶ Healthcare Quality Improvement Partnership | Guide for clinical audit leads

▶ HSJ | Future of NHS leadership

▶ HSJ | Moving from compliance to building a safety culture

▶ Hunter Healthcare | What makes a top chair?

▶ Hunter Healthcare | What makes a top chief executive?

▶ Hunter Healthcare | What makes a top clinical director?

▶ Hunter Healthcare | What makes a top medical director?

▶ Investors in People | 6 questions to help line managers get feedback

▶ Investors in People | 7 tips for a healthier work-life balance

▶ Investors in People | 7 ways HR can help diverse teams succeed

▶ Investors in People | 10 tips for successful succession planning

▶ Investors in People | 11 time management techniques to share with employees

▶ Investors in People | 15 ideas for improving work-life balance and wellbeing

▶ Investors in People | Creativity in the workplace – 7 surprising truths

▶ Investors in People | Employee recognition schemes – Top tips for success

▶ Investors in People | Energy management at work – 6 ways employees can take action

▶ Investors in People | Feeling valued – The dimensions organisations must deliver on

▶ Investors in People | Giving praise – A useful framework managers can follow

▶ Investors in People | Leadership skills – 14 ways to improve them with no money

▶ Investors in People | Line managers – 5 ways to build trust with individuals

▶ Investors in People | Line managers – 5 ways to build trust with teams

▶ Investors in People | Mental wellbeing – 5 work hacks for employees

▶ Investors in People | Mental wellbeing – How HR can help staff manage change

▶ Investors in People | Positive mental wellbeing – How managers can bolster employees

▶ Investors in People | Resilience at work – Get multitasking under control

▶ Investors in People | Top tips for outstanding employee inductions

▶ Investors in People | Using standards to improve performance

▶ Investors in People | Wellbeing at work

▶ Investors in People | What does a no blame culture actually look like?

▶ Investors in People | Work-life balance tips that also make you a better person

▶ Investors in People | Work smarter and live better – Tips for encouraging work-life balance

▶ Jackson, Emily | Medical law

▶ Jones, Bill | British politics

▶ King's Fund | A digital NHS? – An introduction to the digital agenda and plans for implementation

▶ King's Fund | Caring to change – How compassionate leadership can stimulate innovation in health care

▶ King's Fund | Deficits in the NHS

▶ King's Fund | Delivering sustainability and transformation plans

▶ King's Fund | Digital change in health and social care

▶ King's Fund | Embedding a culture of quality improvement
▶ King's Fund | Five big issues for health and social care after the Brexit vote
▶ King's Fund | How health care is funded
▶ King's Fund | Leadership in today's NHS – Delivering the impossible
▶ King's Fund | Leadership needs of medical directors and clinical directors
▶ King's Fund | Leadership vacancies in the NHS
▶ King's Fund | Leading across the health and care system
▶ King's Fund | Making sense of integrated care systems, integrated care partnerships and accountable care organisations in the NHS in England
▶ King's Fund | Making the case for quality improvement – Lessons for NHS boards and leaders
▶ King's Fund | New care models
▶ King's Fund | NHS planning guidance
▶ King's Fund | Organising care at the NHS front line – Who is responsible?
▶ King's Fund | Patient-centred leadership – Rediscovering our purpose
▶ King's Fund | Spending on and availability of health care resources – How does the UK compare to other countries?
▶ King's Fund | Sustainability and transformation plans in the NHS
▶ King's Fund | Talent management – Developing leadership not just leaders
▶ King's Fund | The digital revolution – Eight technologies that will change health and care
▶ King's Fund | The future of leadership and management in the NHS
▶ King's Fund | What are the priorities for health and social care?
▶ King's Fund | What is commissioning and how is it changing?
▶ Kouzes, James; Posner, Barry | Learning leadership – The five fundamentals of becoming an exemplary leader
▶ KPMG | The trillion dollar quest – How the world's best healthcare organisations develop managers and leaders
▶ Lee, Karen | Employment law
▶ Lees, Peter | Medical leadership – Time to grow the evidence
▶ Malone, Charles | The art of delegation
▶ Margulis, Alexander | How to rise to the top … and stay there!
▶ Marr, Bernard | Big data
▶ Matthews, Janice; Matthews, Robert | Successful scientific writing
▶ Maxwell, John | Good leaders ask great questions
▶ Maxwell, John | How successful people lead
▶ Maxwell, John | How successful people think
▶ Merkle, Walter | Risk management in medicine

▶ National Quality Board | Shared commitment to quality

▶ NHS | Live well

▶ NHS Careers | Careers in management

▶ NHS Confederation | Leadership in a matrix

▶ NHS Confederation | New care models and staff engagement – All aboard

▶ NHS Confederation | Taking the value-based agenda forward – The five essential components of value-based approaches to health and care

▶ NHS Confederation | The concise NHS handbook

▶ NHS Confederation | Understanding sustainability and transformation plans

▶ NHS Employers | A social media toolkit for the NHS

▶ NHS Employers | Code of conduct for NHS managers

▶ NHS Employers | Employment checks document cross reference tool

▶ NHS Employers | Improving staff retention – A guide for employers

▶ NHS Employers | Leading a healthy workforce – Engaging board and clinical leaders to take positive action on staff wellbeing

▶ NHS Employers | NHS health and wellbeing framework

▶ NHS Employers | NHS health and wellbeing framework diagnostic tool

▶ NHS Employers | Planning successful international recruitment – A guide for employers

▶ NHS Employers | Raising concerns in the NHS – A guide for staff

▶ NHS Employers | Reward communications guide

▶ NHS Employers | Staff engagement – Maintaining and improving in demanding times

▶ NHS Employers | Strategic reward – Communicating reward to new employees

▶ NHS Employers | Strategic reward – Using reward in recruitment

▶ NHS Employers | Supporting line managers to foster engagement

▶ NHS Employers | The NHS workforce

▶ NHS Employers | Using social media during your NHS career

▶ NHS Employers | Using social media in NHS leadership

▶ NHS Employers | Vital signs – Eight elements of workforce wellbeing

▶ NHS Employers, Skills for Care | People performance management toolkit

▶ NHS England | Five year forward view

▶ NHS England | Next steps on the NHS five year forward view

▶ NHS England | Review into the quality of care and treatment provided by 14 hospital trusts in England – Overview report

▶ NHS England | Serious incident framework

▶ NHS England | The NHS constitution

▶ NHS England | Understanding the new NHS

▶ NHS England, NHS Improvement | NHS operational planning and contracting guidance

▶ NHS Improvement | A just culture guide

▶ NHS Improvement | Aligning improvement with strategic goals

▶ NHS Improvement | Consultant job planning – A best practice guide

▶ NHS Improvement | Creating a vision

▶ NHS Improvement | Developing people – Improving care

▶ NHS Improvement | Developmental reviews of leadership and governance using the well-led framework – Guidance for NHS trusts and NHS foundation trusts

▶ NHS Improvement | Healthcare leadership model

▶ NHS Improvement | Leading improvement

▶ NHS Improvement | Leading improvement framework

▶ NHS Improvement | Never events policy and framework

▶ NHS Improvement | Patient experience improvement framework

▶ NHS Improvement | Reducing reliance on medical locums – A practical guide for medical directors

▶ NHS Improvement | Single oversight framework

▶ NHS Improvement | Support for chairs and non-executives

▶ NHS Improvement | Supporting NHS providers on executive HR issues

▶ NHS Improvement | Toolkit for communications and engagement teams in service change programmes

▶ NHS Improvement | Well-led framework

▶ NHS Improvement, Faculty of Medical Leadership and Management | The medical director's role – A guide for aspiring medical leaders

▶ NHS Improvement, NHS England | Freedom to speak up – Raising concerns (whistleblowing) policy for the NHS

▶ NHS Institute for Innovation and Improvement | Thinking differently

▶ NHS Leadership Academy | Healthcare leadership model – The nine dimensions of leadership behaviour

▶ NHS Leadership Academy | Talent management hub – An online talent management resource for everyone working in the NHS

▶ NHS Leadership Academy | The maximising potential conversation tool

▶ NHS Leadership Academy | The talent management conversation tool

▶ NHS Leadership Academy | What is talent management?

▶ NHS Litigation Authority | NHS Litigation Authority guidance on candour

▶ NHS Resolution | Being a witness in a clinical negligence claim

▶ NHS Resolution | Being a witness in a non-clinical negligence claim

▶ NHS Resolution | Giving evidence at court

▶ NHS Resolution | National Clinical Assessment Service – A guide for healthcare professionals

▶ NHS Resolution | Saying sorry

▶ NHS Scotland | Enabling system transformation and positive patient and staff experience

▶ Nigam, Amit | Multiple and competing goals in organisations – Insights for medical leaders

▶ Nigam, Amit; Gao, Minjie | Future of clinical leadership – The critical role of front-line doctors

▶ Nuffield Trust | Delivering the benefits of digital health care

▶ Nuffield Trust | Improving UK health care

▶ Nuffield Trust | Managing doctors, doctors managing

▶ Nuffield Trust | Managing patient flow and improving efficiencies – The role of technology

▶ Nuffield Trust | The four health systems of the UK – How do they compare?

▶ Nuffield Trust | What will new technology mean for the NHS and its patients?

▶ O'Keeffe, Niamh | Your first 100 days – How to make maximum impact in your new leadership role

▶ Owen, Jo | Myths of leadership

▶ Owen, Jo | The leadership skills handbook

▶ Pardey, David | Introducing leadership

▶ Pincus, Marilyn | Managing difficult people

▶ Pink, Daniel | Drive – The surprising truth about what motivates us

▶ Poole, Jon | Leadership

▶ Professional Standards Authority | Standards for members of NHS boards and clinical commissioning group governing bodies in England

▶ Rossiter, Tony | Effective business writing

▶ Rossiter, Tony | Management basics

▶ Royal College of Nurses | Adult safeguarding – Roles and competencies for health care staff

▶ Royal College of Physicians | Improving teams in healthcare

▶ Royal College of Physicians | Unlocking the potential – Supporting doctors to use national clinical audit to drive improvement

▶ Royal College of Radiologists | Standards for self-assessment of performance

▶ Rubenzer, Bernie | Introduction to medical imaging management

▶ Salonek, Tom | The 100 building blocks for business leadership

▶ Shape of Training | Securing the future of excellent patient care

► Shaw, Rory; Ramachandra, Vino; Lucas, Nuala; Robinson, Neville | Management essentials for doctors

► Sinek, Simon | Start with why – How great leaders inspire everyone to take action

► Skills for Care | Core skills

► Skills for Care | Good and outstanding care guide

► Skills for Care | Leadership qualities framework – Guide for those in governance roles

► Skills for Care | Manager induction standards

► Skills for Care | Recommendations for CQC providers guide

► Skills for Care | The social care manager's handbook – A practical guide for registered managers

► Skills for Care | Values based recruitment and retention guide

► Spurgeon, Peter; Clark, John | Medical leadership – The key to medical engagement and effective organisations

► Stern, Stefan; Cooper, Cary | Myths of management

► Swanwick, Tim; McKimm, Judy | ABC of clinical leadership

► Templar, Richard | The rules of management

► Tilmouth, Tina; Quallington, Jan | Diploma in leadership for health and social care – Level 5

► Toler, Stan | Minute motivators for leaders

► Tracy, Brian | Leadership

► Tracy, Brian | Management

► UK Trade & Investment | Invest in the UK – Your springboard for global growth

► Vincent, Charles; Amalberti, René | Safer healthcare

► Virginia Mason Institute | Creativity cards

► Virginia Mason Institute | Leading 5S

► Virginia Mason Institute | Waste walk exercise

► Wallwork, Adrian | English for academic correspondence and socialising

► Watkin, Sara; Vincent, Andrew | The consultant interview

► Weimann, Edda; Weimann, Peter | High performance in hospital management

► Welch, Ellen | The NHS at 70 – A living history

► Whistleblowing Helpline | Raising concerns at work – Whistleblowing guidance for workers and employers in health and social care

► Wilson, Emery; Perman, Jay; Clawson, Kay | Pearls for leaders in academic medicine

► Work Foundation | Exceeding expectation – The principles of outstanding leadership

► www.consultantmedicalinterview.com | Consultant medical interviews